T0194972

Praise for Tristan Taormino

"The modern American sex guru."

—*Penthouse*

"Tristan Taormino is an inspiration and a sensation. She is literally all over the map, from a recent trip to teach sex ed in Germany, to appearances on HBO's *Real Sex* and *Ricki Lake*, to writing a column in the *Village Voice*, and to authoring numerous books, most notably *The Ultimate Guide to Anal Sex for Women*, which landed her on *Howard Stern*. It's hard to even try to summarize her career, so I won't. Suffice it to say, she has her hands (and other body parts) in just about every area of the sex industry, from writing and editing books, to designing butt plugs, to film and television work, to hands-on sex education, and college lecturing."

—Rachel Kramer Bussel

"Editor Tristan Taormino possesses a simple modus operandi. She blends sex and writing. And like Susie Bright before her, Taormino prepares a potent cocktail."

—Bay Windows Online

"With her soft, chestnut colored curls, 21st-century modified cat-eye glasses, fitted black T-shirt, and fabulous brown suede A-line miniskirt that showcase her creamy skin and alluring tattoos, Taormino is that delightful rarity: a sexy, intellectual post-punk librarian-type who writes columns about getting through heightened airport security with her adult toys after September 11."

—Kera Bolonik, *Hartford Courant*

"As Taormino has shaped her career, her brand of feminism has promoted realistic views of sex and sexuality by keeping politics and ethics at the forefront of her work. She had to carve her own path, but in doing so, she paved the way for dynamic change."

—wesleying.org

50
SHADES
OF KINK

50 SHADES OF KINK

AN INTRODUCTION TO BDSM

TRISTAN TAORMINO

FOREWORD BY RACHEL KRAMER BUSSEL

CLEiS
PRESS

Printed in the United States.
Cover design: Scott Idleman/Blink
Cover photograph: Celesta Danger
Text design: Frank Wiedemann

First Edition.
10 9 8 7 6 5 4 3 2 1

Trade paper ISBN: 978-1-62778-030-8
E-book ISBN: 978-1-57344-940-3

Library of Congress Cataloging-in-Publication Data is available.

CONTENTS

〈〉〉〉〉〉〉〉〉〉〉〉

A LIFELONG LEARNING PROCESS

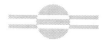

I distinctly remember being uncertain of what to expect—from myself and my fellow partygoers—at my first play party. I was excited, curious, and deeply nervous. I didn't want to say yes to something that I couldn't get out of. I wasn't sure what was going to happen, what exactly I wanted to happen, or even what the options were. This brave new sexy world was thrilling—and more than a little overwhelming.

I've also encountered that same sensation in one-on-one situations, where a part of me is curious about taking a kinky fantasy to the next level, but another part of me is far more hesitant. Quite often, I get off on that mental space in between full abandon and erring on the side of caution, and much of my erotic writing stems from that place. But it's taken a lot of trial and error to figure out exactly where my *yeses, nos*, and *maybes* fall (and to realize they won't always stay the same), to know what I want out of BDSM scenes and relationships, and what I don't. The book you're holding in your hands is one that can help guide you as you figure out what kink is all about, and where you (and/or your partner[s]) fit in.

I was especially pleased to see Tristan tackle this subject with such openness, intelligence, thoroughness, and mindfulness. She gives you all of the good stuff—the ins and outs of dominance and submission, spankings, bondage (and more bondage!), rough sex, and other fun topics—but she also delves deeply into the less "sexy" but equally vital aspects of kink like safe words, limits, and aftercare.

I could have used the very first item on her list of what to carry in your toy bag—consent—along with the second—communication—at a play party

I wound up in the midst of a few years ago. It was one that sprang up seemingly minutes after another event I was attending wrapped up. I wasn't prepared or interested in playing with anyone, but I suddenly found myself holding a rope as part of a scene. Nobody told me exactly what was happening or asked if I wanted to hold this rope; it was thrust in my hand and I was expected to simply follow along. The scene involved someone being bound, and those of us holding onto the ropes were supposed to tighten or loosen them depending on the sub's nonverbal cues. I'd never participated in anything like this and was, frankly, terrified. Only later, once I'd extricated myself, did I realize I was also annoyed. While in another setting, where I would have been part and parcel of the planning of such a scene and known and consented to what was happening, I may very well have been into it; in the real-life version, I wasn't.

Though I should have been smart enough to walk away immediately, there was a part of me that didn't want to let anyone down, or admit weakness. In hindsight, I'm fully aware that turning down a scene or kinky proposition isn't a sign of weakness, but its opposite—strength. It means you know yourself, your desires, and needs enough to stand up for them—and I daresay that will make you a better top, bottom, dom, sub, and/or lover.

That episode taught me that whether you've only dreamt about such a scenario or think you've been there, done that, we could all use some reinforcement of the basics of consent and safety covered in *50 Shades of Kink*. After all, kink isn't a class we're taking pass/fail, with hastily scribbled notes we'll discard the moment we exit the classroom door. Rather, BDSM can be a lifelong learning process and way of getting to know ourselves and our deepest, and sometimes darkest, fantasies and fetishes.

There are things on the "Yes–No–Maybe" list in this book that I would have never even entertained as a nervous newbie at that first play party which now play an active role in my life in some way, whether as a common activity or fodder for dirty talk and fantasy. Those shifts never could have happened without first getting comfortable with my own kinks and learning how they can be practiced safely and erotically. I've funneled many of these fantasies into my erotic fiction, from the desire to be spanked until I cry, to hair pulling, to being "forced" to do various humiliating tasks. Giving free rein to my kinky imagination via erotica has helped me figure out which of those sometimes outlandish, outrageous fantasies work best in theory and which I'd like to try in practice. It's been a safe space to explore and accept the places my mind can go when I know I won't be questioned, or judged, or prompted to act on my curiosity immediately.

All those things I was worried about the first time I lay down across a lover's lap for a spanking, the first time I agree to be tied up in public—and, to be honest, even now—are dealt with in the pages of this book.

All of us at times need to know we're not alone, especially when our sexual fantasies veer down a path that may unnerve, surprise, confuse, or confound us. We may not know what to do with the internal input we're getting about what turns us on. We'll think to ourselves, *But what does it mean that I get off thinking about bukkake, or bondage, or kidnapping, or being a plaything passed around at a party—or, on the other side, being the one holding someone else's deepest desires in the palm of my hand?*

Don't worry—you don't have to know exactly what it all means to know that you are in control of what you do with your newfound (or longtime) curiosity. What you will take away from this expert introduction is a better sense of the right questions to ask yourself as you start or continue your erotic explorations, as well as a glimpse into the many varied twists and turns the journey can take you. Which ones you choose are up to you. The best part? You can keep on choosing, changing, and mixing it up as you go along.

Rachel Kramer Bussel

INTRODUCTION

FIFTY MORE SHADES

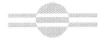

It may have started as *Twilight* fan fiction, but the *Fifty Shades of Grey* trilogy by E. L. James grew quickly into an international phenomenon. The first book in the series is the UK's bestselling book (beating out *Harry Potter*), has been translated into thirty languages, and has sold over forty million copies worldwide so far.

As a sex educator and erotica editor, what excites me most about *Fifty Shades of Grey* is the widespread impact it has made: never before has an erotic novel been responsible for causing such a stir. In addition to driving up the sales of Ben Wa balls, it has captured the imagination of so many different kinds of people and sparked important conversations about desire and power. And there is more widespread interest in kink than ever before.

I use *kink* as a catch-all term that includes BDSM, sadomasochism, kinky sex, dominance and submission, role play, sex games, fantasy, and fetish. But that definition just leads to more terms that need defining! I will both define and expand on these words throughout this book, but for now, if you're reading this, I'll assume you have a basic idea of what I'm talking about.

Beyond definitions, what is kink really? And why do people do it? Kink is an intimate experience, an exchange of power between people that can be physical, erotic, sexual, psychological, spiritual, or, most often, some combination. People who practice kink explore the territory between pleasure and pain, eroticize the exchange of power, experience intense physical sensations and psychological scenarios, and test and push their limits. Kink can be a unique laboratory—a sacred space where we feel safe enough to try new things, push our boundaries, flirt with edges, and conquer fears. Members of BDSM or kink communities emphasize consent above all else—everyone is on board with what's going on and nothing happens against anyone's will. They value trust, communication, and safety, and often make use of a safeword—a word that either partner can use to bring everything to a stop. Kink is one area of the spectrum of sexual practices, so people do kink for as many reasons as people have sex: to give, to take, to connect, to discover, to trust, to experiment, to imagine, to learn, and to grow.

One of the components of the *Fifty Shades of Grey* books that has been widely criticized is its inaccurate representation of kink practices. Many of the details simply don't ring true for those of us who've practiced kink for many years, and additionally, the book portrays some unrealistic and unsafe activities. I realize that it's a romance novel, *fiction*, and was never intended to be an instructional manual of any kind; however, based on media reports and a huge spike in kinky toy sales at sex retailers, lots of readers have been inspired to try out some of the fantasy material in real life. As an educator, I know how important it is for people to have accurate, honest, and straightforward information about sexuality. It was pure luck and coincidence that my own book about kink, *The Ultimate Guide to Kink: BDSM, Role Play and the Erotic Edge*, came out just a few months after *Fifty Shades of Grey* caught fire, and *The Ultimate Guide* has certainly benefitted from the newfound popularity of kink. But I realized quickly that some people were searching for a more basic kinky education, so I wrote this book as a kind of how-to companion to the novels.

This is a primer for people who are interested in kink and want to know more about it, learn how to negotiate with a partner, get some ideas, and explore different activities; it's meant to be an introduction to the world of kink. In it, you'll learn the truth behind common myths about kink, how to talk about your fantasies, common kinky terms and tenets, dominant/submissive role play, and sexual power games. In addition, you'll find ideas, tips, and techniques for different kinky activities, including sensory deprivation, sensation play, bondage, spanking, flogging, and more. If you want to go deeper and find out more, check out my book *The Ultimate Guide to Kink: BDSM, Role Play and the Erotic Edge*, as well as the titles listed in the reading list at the end of this book.

Tristan Taormino

CHAPTER 1

EMBRACE YOUR INNER KINKSTER:
MYTHS, TRUTHS, AND COMMUNICATION

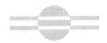

Let's say you read *Fifty Shades of Grey* or another erotic, kinky novel like *Carrie's Story* by Molly Weatherfield or *The Marketplace* by Laura Antoniou. You enjoyed these fictional accounts of dominance and submission, power and lust, pleasure and pain, hot sex and incredible orgasms. You enjoyed them *a lot*. But, perhaps you or your partner have some reservations about these newfound fantasies. Portrayals of kink, a.k.a. BDSM, in the mainstream media—from novels and magazines to television and movies—are generally inaccurate, misleading, one-dimensional, or just plain wrong. As a result, there are a lot of myths about kinky people and practices out there. If you're struggling with some things you read or heard about kink or these concerns are holding you back from exploring your desires, this summary of some of the most popular misconceptions, along with the real facts, should provide you with reassurance, clarity, and support about your fantasies and desires.

Myths about BDSM and Kinky People

◇◇◇◇◇◇◇◇

Myth: BDSM is the same thing as violence and abuse.

Violence and abuse are horrific and should not be tolerated under any circumstances. Some BDSM activities (bondage, slapping, verbal degradation), if they are taken out of their erotic context, may *resemble* violent acts, but they are not at all; they are consensual activities between adults who derive pleasure from them and who have the power to stop the activities at any time.

Myth: If you had a satisfying sex life, your partner wouldn't want to try anything kinky.

If you or your partner has just discovered an interest in kink, it is not an indictment of your current sex life; people's sexual tastes are varied and change over time. If a new desire has emerged, consider it a gift, not a warning sign. People do BDSM for the same wide variety of reasons people have sex, including pleasure and connection. Just as some people love oral sex and others love sex in the woods, some love BDSM. Plenty of folks have told me they believe it's just how they're wired. I've heard countless stories of the first time a lover held her down, the first time a man put a collar on her, the first time she got spanked. Many experienced a visceral reaction to these experiences before they had language to describe what they were doing or knew there were other people out there doing similar things. For some, BDSM does not have to focus on or even involve genital stimulation to be pleasurable and even orgasmic. For

> *If a new desire has emerged, consider it a gift, not a warning sign.*

others, a good flogging and a good fucking is the perfect combination—BDSM enhances the sexual experience.

Myth: Bottoms, submissives, and masochists have low self-esteem or intimacy issues.

Bottoms like to have things done to them. Masochists enjoy intense sensations, including what other people may interpret as pain or discomfort. Submissives want to submit to a partner on their terms. What these roles have in common is that the people who embody them write the script, dictate what they want done to them, and can put a stop to it immediately; they actually have a great deal of power in the situation. Submissives in particular are stereotyped as timid and passive, which misses some of the key elements of the dominant/submissive power dynamic. Submissives generally like the freedom that comes with having

> *It's all about the context of the situation—someone can be very "take charge" in everyday life, but like to be ordered around in bed.*

someone else be in charge; they don't have to think about what comes next or make decisions, they just have to follow a partner's lead. Submission can give some people permission to explore certain sexual desires without guilt or shame ("I have to do everything my master says..."). Some submissives get a thrill from being sexually available to their partner; they don't have to wait for someone to initiate sex or think about the next move. Some enjoy being the center of attention. Others like the opportunity to focus exclusively on their partner's sexual needs over their own, which is a huge turn-on for lots of people. It's all about the context of the situation— someone can be very "take charge" in everyday life, but like to be ordered around in bed.

Myth: Tops, dominants, and sadists are sociopaths who have intimacy issues.

Tops are doers. Dominants like to be the boss. Sadists like to inflict pain and discomfort. Nothing is wrong with any of these desires. These three roles share a common desire to take charge and guide the erotic encounter. Some people prefer to lead in life, and that preference extends to their sexual lives (others may like to express their leadership in bed more than elsewhere). They derive pleasure from being skilled in a particular activity and the ability to bring their partners pleasure. They like to watch as someone becomes putty in their hands, giving in to the experience. What kind of a person wants to hurt their partner? Again, you must return to the context of the scene: sadists inflict pain on folks who *enjoy* the experiences.

Myth: If you enjoy pain, something is wrong with you.

When some people think of activities like flogging, caning, or spanking, they often think of pain. And no one gets turned on by or enjoys pain, right? Actually, some people do. When people experience pain, adrenaline, endorphins, and natural painkillers flood their nervous systems. Some people get off on this chemical rush, which many describe as feeling energized, high, or transcendent. Pain is not just a physical event; like many things in our culture, it is also socially constructed and reinforced. When we see a person slap someone's face, we think, "That hurt, that was unpleasant." But, in the context of a sexually charged scene, when some people are aroused (and their pain tolerance is much higher), they process a face slap in a different way: it feels *good*. They like how their flesh responds and their pulse quickens. It may feel shocking, intimate, stinging; add the taboo of dominance, punishment, humiliation—whatever that slap signifies for those two people—and you've got a recipe for an intense, pleasurable experience. In certain contexts, one person's pain can be another person's pleasure. Or, as Patrick Califia writes in *The Ultimate Guide to Kink*, "Euphoria and agony are next-door neighbors."

Myth: Kinky desires are not normal.

We have to stop thinking of kink as something abnormal or perverse and instead recognize it as part of a broad spectrum of desires. We should not put moral judgments on people who like certain kinds of sex. Imagine if we did that with nonkinky sex. Why does he like the doggie-style position so much? Why doesn't she enjoy receiving oral sex more? Questions like those sound ridiculous, because we accept that some people like this, other people like that,

> *Life's too short to second-guess your desires and what they might mean about you.*

and plenty of people like both. If it turns you on, you're doing it with consenting adults, you're not breaking laws or ruining your own life or someone else's, just stop worrying and go for it. Life's too short to second-guess your desires and what they might *mean* about you.

Myth: Kinky people were abused as children, and they are acting out their abuse.

There is actually no research which supports this myth, yet it persists. Do some kinky people engage in very emotionally and/or physically intense practices? Yes. Do some people get off on being pushed to their limits, seeing how much pain they can take, enduring an intense experience, or exploring dark psychological territory? Yes. In fact, some people do create and enact scenes that echo past traumas in their lives, but there is a major difference between simply repeating past abuse and purpose-fully crafting an erotic scenario in order to experience catharsis and healing. In real trauma, you feel powerless. In the latter, you write the script, you control the scene, and you have the power.

Communicating with Your Partner

The truth behind these myths is an important piece in your own journey of self-discovery and can help you embrace your newfound kinky fantasies. Once you get more comfortable with them, you may begin to imagine some scenes you've read about or watched in a film becoming a part of your real sex life. You think about what it might be like to spank your partner or be someone's sex slave, but how do you begin? First, you need to share your fantasies with your partner, which I realize is sometimes easier said than done. But the only way you will have the opportunity to explore these desires is if you put yourself out there and tell your partner what you really want. Communication is a crucial component of an empowered and fulfilling sex life. There are a number of different ways you can do it, and it all depends on your communication style.

Be direct. The success of the *Fifty Shades of Grey* trilogy has inspired a new open dialogue about kink among many different kinds of people, and the books are a great way to start the conversation. "So, I read this book, and it turned me on, and I'd like to try some of the stuff with you," is about as direct as you can get. While you're being so direct, you can also get specific; you can say, "One of the things in the book that really got me going was [fill in your favorite: bondage, role play, blindfolds, candles, etc.]." You

> *Communication is a crucial component of an empowered and fulfilling sex life.*

can also talk about how you might like something different: "In the book, Christian uses a riding crop on Anastasia's vulva, but I think I'd like you to try using it on my butt cheeks instead." Give your partner the space to listen, and tell him he does not have to respond right away if he doesn't want to. If beginning that directly scares you, try the following techniques first and work your way up to a more explicit discussion.

Write it down. If talking about your desires face-to-face with your partner makes you feel shy, intimidated, or overwhelmed, you could write her a note. Handwritten notes are a rarity these days, so it should get his attention. You can use the same direct approach, but put it on paper, then slip the note to her. Or you can email him a note (as long as it's not to a work email account!). Sending a handwritten or emailed note gives you a chance to compose your thoughts and takes any pressure off the situation; it gives her the opportunity to digest the new information and respond when she's ready. As a bonus, it could spark a series of erotic notes you write back and forth to each other about exactly what you want to do together.

> *If you're not quite sure how to express your desires, let the book that inspired you do it for you.*

Use the book. If you're not quite sure how to express your desires, let the book that inspired you do it for you. Select some of your favorite passages and print out or photocopy those pages, highlight the particularly incendiary sections, and include them with your note. Bonus points for under-lining, color coding certain activities, writing in the margins, or creating your own footnotes.

Chat in cyberspace. Sometimes you feel a little bolder if you aren't sitting in the same room with your partner, so try chatting online with instant messages. Unlike email, this gives you the chance to have a real-time dialogue, but there is still a little distance, which may increase your bravery. You can begin the conversation the same way, "I read this book…" and take it from there. This will give your partner a chance to ask questions and you a chance to be specific. Chatting online can also be a way to start the discussion that can then continue in person later.

Go shopping. Take a trip to your local sex toy store and head to the fantasy role play or bondage section. You both can point out toys that interest you, talk about who wants to do what with them. You don't actually have to buy anything; you can simply use the selection of implements to start the conversation, give you ideas, and point out your preferences. Or you can make a purchase that becomes the spark for your new erotic adventure.

A movie will give you a visual encyclopedia of different activities, power dynamics, and scenarios—use that information to begin to talk about what you want to do.

Watch a movie. Pick an adult film with similar themes to a book you like; *O: The Power of Submission* directed by Ernest Greene, for example, is a modern-day retelling of Pauline Réage's book *Story of O* (see sidebar for more recommendations). As you watch it together, chime in about what interests you, what turns you off, and what you find intriguing but you're not sure you're ready to try. A movie will give you a visual encyclopedia of different activities, power dynamics, and scenarios—use that information to begin to talk about what you want to do.

Inspiration on Film:
Great BDSM Porn Films

❋ ❋ ❋ ❋ ❋

O: The Power of Submission (Adam & Eve)

The Surrender of O (Adam & Eve)

The Truth About O (Adam & Eve)

The *Rough Sex* series (Vivid)

The Fashionistas (Evil Angel)

The *Fetish Fanatic* series (Evil Angel)

Nina Hartley's Guide to Erotic Bondage (Adam & Eve)

Midori's Expert Guide to Sensual Bondage (Vivid-Ed)

Penny Flame's Expert Guide to Rough Sex (Vivid-Ed)

Tristan Taormino's Guide to Bondage for Couples (Adam & Eve)

Tristan Taormino's Guide to Kinky Sex for Couples (Adam & Eve)

Crash Pad Series Volume 4: Rope Burn (Pink and White Productions)

The Curse of MacBeth (Madison Bound)

Tail of a Bondage Model (Madison Bound)

50 Shades: A XXX Adaptation (Smash Pictures)

All of these approaches should eventually lead to a frank conversation, one you come to with an open mind, patience, and some information. If your partner has questions, be prepared with answers. Be ready to counteract myths, stereotypes, and misinformation (with assistance from the first part of this chapter).

Sex can be very strongly connected to our egos and our core sense of self; it often makes us feel more vulnerable than anything else we do. It's difficult, especially if you are in a long-term relationship, to reveal that you have a new desire, especially one that's different than what you've expressed in the past. If you realize that going in to the conversation, you will be better prepared for different reactions from your partner which could range from surprise, confusion, and curiosity to shock, hurt, and even anger—or some combination of these. Don't get defensive. Be ready to reassure your partner that this new information doesn't change how you feel about him. Emphasize that these fantasies excite and arouse you, and you want to share that excitement and arousal with him. If you're the one who's hearing this new information, be open. Don't rush to judgment, get defensive, or shut down. Listen to your partner, ask questions, give yourself time to digest the information, and don't feel like you have to respond immediately. Ideally, talking about your fantasies will spark new adventures in bed and bring you closer together.

What If I Don't Have a Partner?

◇◇◇◇◇◇◇◇

When someone expresses an interest in kink, I always give the same advice: find your local community. You can begin online by joining one of the largest kinky social networking sites, FetLife.com, and from there find other online groups and lists that are tailored to your specific interests, identities, experience level, or geographic area. Want to know where the kinksters are in your neighborhood? Google BDSM and your town,

> *Talking about your fantasies will spark new adventures in bed and bring you closer together.*

city, or county, and you'll likely come up with social events, workshops, support groups, conferences, and, for lucky folks, play parties, dungeons, and clubs. There are hundreds of gatherings of kinksters throughout North America and the world—whether a regional organization's annual conference, a camping event for pervy people, or a BDSM retreat—and the majority of them have a strong educational component. On any given weekend, you can learn how to safely set someone on fire, be a good Daddy, plan the perfect orgy, or do bondage without rope.

CHAPTER 2

BDSM BASICS:
TERMS, ROLES, AND PRINCIPLES

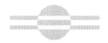

Once you've talked about your kinky desires with your partner, there are a few more aspects to discuss including different roles, activities, and limits. In the spirit of direct communication and clarity, I'd first like to define some terms you will read throughout this book.

Terminology

Kink is an umbrella term for BDSM, kinky sex, dominance and submission, erotic role play, fantasy, and fetish.

BDSM is an acronym and an umbrella term that was first used in the late 80s and early 90s in Internet discussion groups and was more widely adopted in the 2000s. *BDSM* is a combination of several shorter acronyms that reflect the history of our kinky vocabulary and the wide variety of practices that it incorporates:

B & D (also *B/D*) stands for bondage and discipline. It is an older term that first appeared in personals and magazines in the 1970s and became widely used by kinky folks in the 1980s to describe their interest in kink. It wasn't necessarily meant to denote *only* bondage and discipline, but rather a range of activities that revolved around power exchange. Today *B & D* is much less frequently used as a term on its own.

SM (also *S & M*, *S/M*, *S/m*) is the common abbreviation for sadism and masochism or sadomasochism. (See below for definitions of these and related words.) These terms were coined by Richard von Krafft-Ebing in 1886 and have appeared frequently since then in psychoanalytic literature to describe sexual pathologies; however, kinky people reclaimed them beginning around the 1970s, and *SM* was the most popular term for kink activities until *BDSM* gained widespread use by the 2000s.

Sadomasochism is the enjoyment of giving or receiving pain or discomfort.

A *sadist* derives pleasure from inflicting pain, intense sensations, and discomfort on someone else. That pain or discomfort can be phys-

> **SM *was the most popular term for kink activities until* BDSM *gained widespread use by the 2000s.***

ical (like during a spanking), emotional and psychological (as in an interrogation scene), or both.

A *masochist* is someone who enjoys receiving pain or intense sensations, being made uncomfortable, or being "forced" to do something they don't want to do. Remember that sadists and masochists experience these desires and pleasures in the context of consensual BDSM scenes.

D/s (also *DS* or *d/s*) stands for dominance and submission or dominant/submissive. The terms dominant, submissive, and dominance/submission have been around for a long time; people began using them in the context of kink in the 1980s to describe the power dynamic within a SM scene or relationship, or to communicate their interest in roles like master/slave or daddy/boy. In a D/s relationship today, the power exchange may exist without other elements of BDSM.

When a D/s power exchange is always or very often present, partners inhabit their roles and reinforce the dynamic through various rituals, protocols, and behaviors all the time; these relationships may be referred to as *24/7 D/s* (as in 24 hours a day, 7 days a week), *lifestyle D/s*, *TPE* (total power exchange), or *APE* (absolute power exchange). (Read more about dominants and submissives in the next section on roles.)

> **A scene *is where two or more people come together to do BDSM.***

22

BDSM can be used as a noun ("I'm interested in BDSM") or an adjective ("I went to a BDSM event"). Some people use other terms interchangeably with BDSM, including SM, kink, and leather.

The use of the term *leather* in association with BDSM (as in, "I'm part of the local leather community") originated in post-World War II gay male biker clubs and bars and continued in leather bars and sex clubs from the late 50s all the way through the 2000s. *Leather* is still used today, especially by gay, lesbian, bisexual, transgender, and queer folks, to signify kinky interests, identities, and communities.

Play is a common term used to describe the practice of BDSM, as in, "I want to play with a bondage expert so I can learn more about it." It can also be used as an adjective: "My play partner caned me really well at Susan's play party. I'm glad I set up that play date!"

A *scene* is where two or more people come together to do BDSM. People may also use *scene* to describe the BDSM community ("Is she in the scene?"). You can do a scene anywhere, but often people do them in a play space or dungeon. These spaces may be private, such as a room in someone's home, or public, like a large club. Such places often

> One of the first things to consider as you talk about what kinds of BDSM activities you might like to try is what role you'll take in a scene: do you want to be in charge or do you want your partner to be in charge (or both)?

have different stations that feature various types of equipment for BDSM play, such as a St. Andrew's cross (a large X, usually made of wood, with places to attach wrist and ankle cuffs), a bondage bed, a spanking bench, a sling, a medical exam table, and a cage.

Erotic role play (or *fantasy role play*) occurs when you and a partner (or partners) create characters and scenarios to act out fantasies with a sexual component.

The term *fetish* has several meanings. When the word first appeared, *fetish* was a psychological term to denote a particular object that one needed in order to experience sexual pleasure and orgasm. Over time, the word has evolved into a kind of shorthand. Now people use it as a way to describe their favorite kinks, as in a shoe fetish, a foot fetish, a cigar fetish, or an ass fetish. In addition, some people say, "I belong to the fetish scene," meaning they like to dress up in latex, leather, and PVC, and attend fetish parties and balls, but they don't necessarily belong to the local BDSM or leather scene.

Roles

One of the first things to consider as you talk about what kinds of BDSM activities you might like to try is what role you'll take in a scene: do you want to be in charge or do you want your partner to be in charge (or both)? A *top* is the doer who initiates activities and actions and does things to the bottom. Do you love the idea of blindfolding your partner, tying him up, or spanking him? If you like doing things to your partner and want your partner to receive, you will probably enjoy taking on the top role.

A *bottom* follows the top's lead, receives stimulation from the top, and has things done to him or her. If you fantasize about giving control to your partner, being put in bondage, or being whipped, then you should explore the bottom role.

Top and bottom can also be used as verbs, as in "I topped my girlfriend last night." A *switch* is someone who enjoys playing both roles. Whether a switch becomes a top or a bottom can change from one scene to the next; switches may take on a particular role based on the partner they play with or the activity. They can also switch between both roles within one scene.

A *dominant* is the partner in charge; dominants run the show and call the shots. Think of the dominant as the authority figure who should be obeyed. A female dominant is sometimes referred to as a *dominatrix*. A *submissive* is someone who enjoys surrendering to their partner, likes to prioritize the dominant's needs and desires, and gets turned on by being told what to do. Read more about dominant/submissive role play in the next chapter.

People of all different genders are tops,

> **Consent**—*explicit, informed verbal approval after negotiation, a confident and secure "Yes!"—is the bedrock of sex and relationships, and one of the most significant elements of kink.*

bottoms, switches, dominants, and submissives. In this book, I will use "he," "she," "her," and "his" not to proscribe certain roles to certain genders or assume a specific kind of dynamic, but rather to mix it up randomly.

Useful Concepts

◇◇◇◇◇◇◇

Kinky folks have adopted a set of principles that represent some important core values: consent, communication, negotiation, education, safety and risk reduction, and aftercare.

Consent

◇◇◇◇◇◇◇◇

Consent—explicit, informed verbal approval after negotiation, a confident and secure "Yes!"—is the bedrock of sex and relationships, and one of the most significant elements of kink. It's what separates kink from abuse. You will read about consent repeatedly in this book. Securing consent from a partner is a necessity, and this holds true whether the person is brand-new to you, you've played together more than a dozen times, or you've been in a relationship for ten years. Never assume anything. When you ask for consent, you clearly speak your part in the exchange: I need to know you've agreed to this before we begin. Giving your consent to a partner prior to a scene is absolutely crucial. It establishes that you're ready, willing, and able to proceed; you've discussed what's likely to happen, shared any concerns, talked about your limits, and agreed to dive in. When you give consent, you do so willingly, without pressure, coercion, or reservation. You agree to play, communicate during the scene, and stop if you need to.

Communication and Negotiation

Giving your consent and receiving a partner's consent is part of the process of negotiating a kink scene. *Negotiation* creates a space for everyone to talk about their needs, wants, limits, fantasies, and fears before they play. One way to begin the negotiation process is to identify what role or roles you will take on: top/bottom/switch, dominant/submissive, sadist/masochist. Together you can discuss possible activities; for each one, you can decide if you are interested in doing it and whether you want to give or receive or both.

BDSM encompasses so many different activities, turn-ons, fetishes, and scenarios that listing them all would take up way too much space here. Plus, there can never be a complete list, since folks are coming up with new kinks every day. Many lists of kinks can be found on the Internet, such as the kinky social networking site FetLife.com, where you'll find a list of thousands of different kinks. Sites like FetLife are also good places to virtually meet others who enjoy BDSM, including people who can act as mentors as you explore the world of kink.

Checklists

◇◇◇◇◇◇◇◇

> **If you get to know your partner better and it feels right, you'll go for it.**

People sometimes make a "Yes–No–Maybe" checklist, marking *yes* for the things they'd like to do, *no* for the things they definitely don't want to do, and *maybe* for activities that fall in between. These lists help you think about what you want to try (or not) as well as assist you in communicating that information to your partner—and vice versa.

The *maybe* list is the trickiest to define, since it's often made up of activities that fall into a grey area; a "maybe" can have multiple meanings. Here are some reasons why you might check *maybe*:

- You are curious about an activity but have no idea if you'll like it.
- You want to find out more information before you mark it with a *yes* or *no*.
- If you and/or your partner became skilled at doing it, then you'd give it a go.

- Once you have more experience with other activities, you may want to try *this* activity.
- It doesn't warrant a *yes*, but you aren't opposed to trying it.
- This activity both excites you and scares you, so you're not sure what to do.
- If you get to know your partner better and it feels right, you'll go for it.
- If you learn to get over your anxiety about it, it could become a *yes*.
- Under the right circumstances, you might like to do it.
- You've never thought about it, but your gut doesn't say *no*.

Talking openly about why something ends up in the *maybe* column will give your partner insight and information about your desires, so be as open as you can.

This book is meant to be a primer for kink, so I'm going to list some of the most popular kinks suited best for beginners to this kind of erotic play. After you read the chapters that follow, which discuss these

activities in more detail, come back to this checklist
and talk to your partner about each entry.

Sample Checklist

◇◇◇◇◇◇◇◇

ACTIVITY	YES	NO	MAYBE	COMMENTS
spanking				
paddle				
crop				
cane				
slapping				
flogging				
blindfold				
ball/mouth gag				
DIY bondage				
restraints				

bondage tape				
rope bondage				
hot wax				
sensation play				
nipple clamps				
hair pulling				
biting				
scratching				
collar				
leash				
dom/sub roles				
pleasure/orgasm control				

Note: this list is just the beginning. Other popular kink activities not on this list include clips and clamps, bondage with suspension, genitorture, mummification, face slapping, animal role play, age play, taboo play, mindfuck, objectification, medical play, electricity play, play piercing/temporary piercing, singletail whipping, and many more. If you want to learn more about these and other more advanced BDSM activities, read my book *The Ultimate Guide to Kink: BDSM, Role Play and the Erotic Edge.*

In addition to negotiating your wants, needs, desires, and limits for BDSM, you should also decide if there will be sexual activity as part of your play. You can write up a similar "Yes–No–Maybe" list for this kind of contact. Will there be genital touch and stimulation? Masturbation? How about penetration, oral sex, sex toys, ejaculation? As part of the negotiation process, you should also disclose when you were last tested for sexually-transmitted infections (STIs) and decide on safer-sex practices.

Making a list of activities is like drawing the outline. Now it's time to fill in the details and get more specific. Erotic desire is in the details, so it will be helpful to you and your partners to flesh out your fantasies and figure out exactly what you want. Say you like the idea of bondage. Do you crave being restrained into submission or do you like the idea of struggling to get out of it? Perhaps you enjoy dominating. Do you prefer to give orders, create predicaments, or use someone for your pleasure? You know you're into sex-for-money fantasies where you're a prosti-tute—but are you a streetwalking hustler or a high-priced call girl?

> *Erotic desire is in the details.*

As you fill in the details of your desires, decide on and communicate your limits within a certain activity, like these:

- You love to be slapped and spanked, but not on your face.
- You're excited to have hot wax dripped on you, but you don't want it on your breasts.
- You checked *yes* under clips and clamps, but you have one caveat: no clothespins.

- You're game to try sensory deprivation if your partner promises not to put a gag in your mouth.
- Caning is fun, but no marks on your body that people could see when you wear shorts.

Now is also the time to tell your partner all relevant information he should know about you. Is there anything in your medical history that is serious or will affect the type of play you do? You should let a partner know if you have a heart condition, high blood pressure, diabetes, allergies, or similar ailments. You should talk about medications you take, a sensitivity to hot or cold, if you're prone to dizziness or fainting, how well you can see without your glasses. Do you have bad knees and can't kneel for more than twenty minutes? That is vital information to tell a dominant before a scene!

> *You should also share any specific elements that you know can trigger a negative reaction in you.*

Although it can be difficult, you should also share any specific elements that you know can trigger a negative reaction in you; these may be based on phobias, negative experiences, past trauma, childhood abuse, or strong aversions. They can be about a specific body part, an activity, an implement, a certain word or words. I have a friend who cannot be spanked with a hairbrush because she has awful memories of being punished as a little girl with a hairbrush by her mother. Another friend likes to be called names like *whore* or *bitch* in a scene but draws the line at *cow* or *pig*. I know a guy who has an intense fear of being strangled, so even hands around his neck can send him into a tailspin. One woman had a bad first-time experience with nipple clamps, and now they give her tremendous anxiety.

This is important information to know as you decide if you're going to play with someone, what you're going to do, and how to construct a scene. This information sharing is part of giving and receiving *informed* consent; it also helps prepare you to assess the risks and determine how to play safer.

Education

◇◇◇◇◇◇◇◇

Education is a very important part of the BDSM community, and you'll find that there is a wide variety of ways to learn kinky skills including educational books, videos, websites, classes, and events. If you're interested in spanking, flogging, sensory deprivation, or acting as a top in any other BDSM activities with a partner, it's important that you learn how to do them correctly from experienced people first. Investigate your local community to see if there is an organization that hosts classes or weekend events. Learning about proper techniques, common mistakes, safety issues, and risk reduction tips will provide you with a solid foundation. And educational classes are not just for tops; there are classes for bottoms where you can learn about negotiating skills, pain processing, and other useful information. After that, it's all about practice!

Safety, Risk, and Responsibility

The issues of safety and responsibility have been vital for kinky people both personally and politically. People who practice BDSM have long emphasized the importance of mentoring and education so newcomers can learn proper skills before picking up a paddle or a flogger. From the time when SM groups first became visible, and as they have continued to grow and become more politically active, kinksters have always wanted nonkinky folks to know that they aren't whip-toting lunatics.

Coined in the 1980s by an SM activist group, the phrase "safe, sane, and consensual" is a concept many kinksters embrace—it prioritizes a commitment to consent and both physical and psychological safety. Others prefer "risk-aware consensual kink" (RACK). RACK also emphasizes the consensual nature of BDSM while acknowledging that some of its practices are inherently risky (and, in fact, exploring the risks and edges are part of what draws people to them). You can make an informed decision to acknowledge the risks, take steps to reduce them, and proceed.

One way to reduce risk is to use a *safeword*. Although you negotiate and discuss

> **Your safeword is your safety net.**

limits, boundaries, and triggers before a scene, you cannot prepare for everything. It's simply impossible to predict how you'll feel during a scene, what will push your buttons, or how something will affect you.

A *safeword* is a word—usually one that you wouldn't normally utter during sex or a scene—that you and your partner choose in advance. Your safeword is your safety net. If you don't like something that's happening and you want the scene to stop right away, simply say your safeword. Words like *stop* or *no* or *please don't*, which we commonly use to communicate this sentiment in day-to-day life, may be part of the dialogue of a BDSM scene where the bottom wants to resist or be forced to do something. So *stop*, *no*, and the like are not ideal safewords. The most common safeword is *red*. Sometimes people pick two different words; one pair often used together are *red* and *yellow*, where red means "stop right now!" and yellow means "please slow down." If the bottom can't speak (he has a gag in his mouth or she is supposed to perform oral sex until you tell her to stop) or the music is really loud in the dungeon, agree on a *safe signal* instead. One such signal is to have the bottom hold something in her hand during a scene, like a tennis ball; if she drops it, that means stop.

Another way to reduce risk is to know what you're doing. As I mentioned earlier, there is a tremendous emphasis on education in the BDSM community, so take advantage of the resources around you. Learn proper techniques, ask fellow practitioners, attend classes and demonstrations by BDSM educators, and practice skills under the guidance of someone experienced. Learn the risks, the common mistakes that people make, and what is most likely to go wrong. The chance to get some hands-on practice with an experienced person is even better. Don't get tipsy or do drugs, then decide to try out your new flogger. Beginning BDSM play is just like lots of things in life: cut yourself some slack. Give each other the benefit of the doubt. Use common sense.

Feedback

◇◇◇◇◇◇◇◇◇◇

During a scene, communication can be more of a challenge. Certainly you could do a scene where you speak freely and give your partner feedback, like this:

- Can you slow down a little?
- Oh, the cane stings more on my thighs than my butt.
- How does this flogger feel compared to the one I just used on you?
- I really like the needles in my chest.
- That dildo's too big. Do you have the blue one?
- You reacted a lot more when the wax came close to your neck.
- Shall I adjust the nipple clamps? Can you take them just a little tighter?

But there may be circumstances that prevent this kind of open dialogue. If you're striving to maintain a strong D/s dynamic in the scene, then a submissive's feedback needs to be more cleverly solicited and spoken. In fact, you can reinforce the power dynamic using words. Have the submissive ask for each slap of your hand, count each stroke of the cane, or even beg for the next drop of hot wax. Instruct the submissive to add some *pleases* and *thank yous* after each drop or make him count each paddle strike. Not only does this move the scene along nicely, it gives the submissive the opportunity to communicate his state of mind. If he begins to wince or hesitate as he speaks, he may be nearing his limit.

Similarly, if you're in a role-playing scene, you want to stay in role. A student doesn't say to the teacher, "Do

> *In fact, you can reinforce the power dynamic using words.*

it harder!" just as a victim doesn't tell his attacker, "Please slow down." Or maybe a bottom wants to be taken on a journey, and neither of you want there to be a lot of back-and-forth chat. You want to lose yourself in the rhythm of the flogging, the sensation of the paddle against your skin, or the feet you plan to worship before you. In some kinds of scenes, a

bottom is flying so high
that she slips into deep
subspace, a trancelike
state some bottoms can
achieve, especially in

> *If you're in a role-playing scene, you want to stay in role.*

a heavy scene, that often leaves them incoherent.
In these situations, eye contact and nonverbal
communication are critical. As a top, your ability
to read your bottom's body language is essential.
Pay attention to the bottom's breathing rate, facial
expressions, how her body reacts to sensation, and
whether the reaction changes. Use your judgment
about whether something should continue, ratchet
up, or wind down.

Aftercare

◇◇◇◇◇◇◇

What happens after a scene is just as significant as
what goes on during it. Think about it: you've just
had an intimate experience with someone, and you
need to make sure you are both all right physically
and mentally. Whether you play like you have in

the past, do something for the first time, explore a new dynamic, or push harder than ever before, it's wise to check in with each other. A scene is like an extraordinary date, a high-flying adventure, or a one-of-a-kind experience—one or both of you are likely to be flooded with endorphins afterward. You might feel energized and excited, worn out and beat down, or, seemingly inexplicably, both. You may be lightheaded, feel like you've run a marathon, or seen God. You may feel exuberant, meditative, vulnerable, anxious, giddy, confused, scared, transcendent, or dumbfounded at what just happened. These sensations are all completely normal and quite common. Let the feelings, even the scary or overwhelming ones, wash over you. Take a deep breath.

Imagine you've doled out a heavy caning that tested the limits of your partner's body, pain tolerance, stamina, and perseverance. You just gave it, and good—now take care of the person who took it. If you're the top, part of your responsibility is to ensure the well-being of your bottom. First address some basic needs with questions like these: do you need to use the bathroom? Do you want to stand up (or sit down—if your bottom has been kneeling or standing during a scene)? Do you want to leave the play space and go somewhere more private, quieter, more comfortable? Are you too warm or too cold? Do you need a blanket

> *As part of your negotiation process, you should discuss any specific needs you both might have after a scene.*

or change of clothes? Offer water or another beverage to make sure the bottom stays hydrated and a snack to combat low blood sugar, especially if the scene involved heavy physical play. As part of your negotiation process, you should discuss any specific needs you both might have after a scene. That way, you can come prepared rather than scrambling to find an energy bar or a sweatshirt for someone who needs it right away.

Some partners want to process their experiences and feelings about the scene right away, so you need to be prepared to do that; people may have a lot of different emotions afterward. Be ready to listen, validate, and comfort. Some people want sex play, making out, or some sweet cuddling as part of aftercare. Others just need a few kind words, a hug, and a lollipop, and they're on their way. After an intense scene, it is a good idea to follow up with a check-in a day or two later; often right after a scene, you're still in the afterglow, but later, feelings may come up that you want to discuss. *Bottom drop* is a common experience where, after the high of a scene wears off (which can take hours or days), a bottom suddenly feels sad, depressed, anxious, lonely, or confused. The antidote if you experience this drop is often to reach out to partners, friends, and loved ones for support and reassurance.

> **Be ready to listen, validate, and comfort.**

Since the bottom is the one who receives the cane strikes, the piercing needles, or the interrogation, there is often a lot of emphasis on the bottom's safety, comfort, and well-being. Do not forget that tops (and dominants and sadists) also need safewords, have limits, and want aftercare. Tops: make sure you take care of yourself, have what you may need handy, and ask for what you want. Postscene, tops may experience the malaise of *top drop*, and anyone can encounter *event drop*, which frequently happens after you get home from a fun, play-filled BDSM event. Aftercare is different for everyone; don't assume you know what someone wants—ask.

Contracts

Contracts are a great way to articulate your needs, wants, limits, and boundaries. Writing a contract can help both partners think carefully about what they want, what they expect, and what they are willing to commit to. Putting it all down on paper can often clarify each partner's position in a concrete way. All that said, a contract is not *necessary* to practice BDSM with someone. What *is* necessary is communication and negotiation, and a contract can

> *Most people have very short contracts, then they renegotiate as they get to know each other better and figure out what works and what doesn't.*

capture all that in writing. Don't think of a contract as a legal document, think of it as an erotic agreement. Don't ever use the contract as a weapon or to excuse bad behavior ("But it didn't say anything about that in our contract…"). If you're interested in writing a contract, here are some points you can consider addressing:

- each person's role
- your goals—what you want to get out of the BDSM exchange or relationship
- each person's physical, psychological, and emotional limits; you could also include the entire "Yes–No–Maybe" list in the contract
- each person's safeword(s)
- rules you've both agreed to
- when and where these roles, rules, and the behavior that accompanies them are in effect (during a scene, at kinky parties and events, in the house when the kids are asleep, or in the bedroom only)

- how long the contract is for; you could do a contract for one day, one week, or several months. If someone you just met asks you to sign a contract of a year or more, that should be a red flag. Most people have very short contracts, then they renegotiate as they get to know each other better and figure out what works and what doesn't.

Sample Contract

❖ ❖ ❖ ❖ ❖

This document is intended to specify the respon-sibilities of [Person 1] (hereafter "the dominant") and [Person 2] (hereafter "the submissive") as part of a consensual arrangement between them. This agreement is valid until midnight on [DATE]. This contract is a private agreement between the parties and it is to be read by only the dominant and the submissive.

1. The submissive shall devote herself, in mind, body, and spirit to the desires of the dominant. The submissive shall willingly obey him without question, knowing that he will never knowingly subject her to anything that will cause her harm. While in his presence, the submissive shall focus her complete attention, devotion, and service to the dominant.

2. When the submissive is in the presence of the dominant, she shall speak to him with respect and address him as [chosen honorific: Master, Mistress, Ma'am, Sir, etc.] at all times. This respect

shall extend to speaking *of* him as well. She shall address him to all other people, at all times when appropriate, as [chosen honorific: Master, Mistress, Ma'am, Sir, etc.] or *my dominant.*

3. When the submissive is in the presence of the dominant in his home, in a private location, or at a BDSM event, she shall wear the collar he gave her at all times. The collar shall symbolize his dominance over her and her devotion to him.

4. The dominant agrees to attend to the physical, emotional, and mental well-being of the submissive. To enable him to do so, the submissive will answer any question put to her as clearly and honestly as she is able.

5. The submissive will strive to maintain her health and vitality to better serve the dominant. The submissive agrees to notify the dominant of any physical discomfort or illness which may impact the submissive's service.

6. The submissive agrees to make her body available to the dominant whenever, wherever, and however he wishes. The dominant accepts full responsibility for the submissive's safety.

7. The dominant agrees to abide by the boundaries and limits set forth in the submissive's limits list [attached]. Both parties understand that such a list is subject to change; it is the submissive's sole responsibility to inform the dominant of any changes to the list. Moreover, the submissive pledges to try her best to expand her boundaries and limits while in service to the dominant.

8. The dominant agrees that he will make no marks on the submissive's body on the chest, neck, face, or forearms.

9. The dominant and the submissive acknowledge that the safeword to stop an activity is red, and the safeword to slow something down is yellow.

10. When the submissive is in the presence of the dominant, she shall ask permission to do the following: [to speak to the dominant or another person, to leave the presence of the dominant, to go to the bathroom, to eat or drink, to go to sleep, to touch the dominant (unless the dominant specifically instructs her to do so), to touch herself, to have an orgasm, etc.].

11. When the submissive is in the presence of the dominant, she shall have in her possession the following items: [collar, massage oil, lube, condoms, latex gloves, toys, etc.].

12. Should she displease the dominant in any way, the submissive agrees to submit to any punishment that the dominant deems necessary. Punishments will be for the betterment of the submissive only and shall not be undertaken in anger by the dominant.

13. Within forty-eight (48) hours of the expiration of this contract, the dominant and submissive shall negotiate and decide by consensus

to renew the contract for a similar or longer period of time. Either party has the right to amend any part of the contract *before* it is signed. Either party has the right to make the contract null and void but must first contact the other party with a reasonable explanation.

CHAPTER 3

DOMINANT/SUBMISSIVE ROLE PLAY

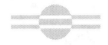

I think I have the classic "businessman syndrome," where being in control all the time and having to make decisions all the time makes you crave someone else's control and want to submit. For me it is very freeing to know that my only obligation is to please someone else. Usually I am the one in charge of everything. It's great to have someone doing that for me.

—DONNA

> *I enjoy being restrained but my preference is to be held down by human force; I like the feeling of hands squeezing my wrists and a knee on my chest, a hard palm pushing on my face. I also enjoy being called names and told that I am only good for fucking and for giving the other person pleasure. Something about being used makes me feel really hot and confident and empowered. Feeling out of control when there is trust and desire involved takes me to a transcendent place that I don't get to on my own or during non-BDSM sex.*
>
> —DYLAN

Role Play

Erotic role play (also called fantasy role play) gives folks a chance to be someone else, even if it's only for an hour or two. You can shake off your real-life self, say a stern, responsible school principal, and become

> *Erotic role play almost always has a power dynamic built right into it.*

someone different, like a pampered princess with a doting babysitter. Role play creates a space for fantasy and make-believe, where you can explore your inner cocky jock, naughty schoolgirl, or bored-but-horny housewife. It can add another layer to your sex life, where you explore the many facets of your own personality, different dynamics with a partner, sexual taboos, and scenarios limited only by your imagination.

Erotic role play almost always has a power dynamic built right into it. Think about some of the most common role-play scenarios: doctor/patient, teacher/student, cop/civilian, prostitute/client. Often these scenes revolve around one person submitting to another, being forced to do something, or feeling vulnerable. Think of a naughty student spanked by a ruler-wielding nun, a professional dominatrix humiliating her client, or a drill sergeant putting a private through his paces. For many people, a significant part of their BDSM play is erotic role play that involves dominance and submission.

Dominance and Submission

<><><><><><><>

In dominant/submissive role play, the *dominant* runs the show, exerts control over a submissive, and may direct him or her to complete tasks, behave a certain way, follow rules, or submit to various kinds of SM (like spanking, bondage, etc.). A *submissive* gives up control and surrenders to the dominant, complies with a dominant's wishes, follows orders, and has an investment in pleasing his or her dominant.

A power exchange of some kind is nearly always present in human relationships. There are people all around us in power exchange relationships who don't acknowledge the dynamic or call it anything. Consider a husband who gives his wife an allowance but no credit card in her own name. A woman who controls her coworkers, making them eager to please her even though she's not their boss. That's right—there are plenty of people wearing collars and others tugging at their leashes, but the gear is invisible and the dynamic unexamined. Kinky people do the opposite: they consciously *create* and *name* a power dynamic in order to eroticize it. By making the power exchange explicit, they get to act on it, play with it, and let it drive the erotic interaction. That exchange is what fuels their desire and pleasure. Think about the mistress who forces her slave to be sexually available to her at all times. Or the submissive who strives to please her dominant, putting his needs above her own.

Service is one kind of D/s dynamic or relationship where the submissive serves the dominant; the dominant may direct the submissive to do household chores, provide sexual stimulation, or complete projects. In fact, ordinary activities that most people take for granted—making

> *Many tops are dominant—their needs and wishes come first—and many bottoms are submissive—their desire is to please and serve their top.*

coffee, drawing a bath, folding laundry—can be imbued with a different meaning and become symbols of submission and service. Service is most often equated with submissives (slaves, boys, girls, etc.), but there are also self-identified *service tops*, who enjoy doing things to bottoms at the bottom's request.

Many tops are dominant—their needs and wishes come first—and many bottoms are submissive—their desire is to please and serve their top. However, that is not always the case. If a dominant master orders his submissive to flog him, then the master is the flogging bottom and the submissive is the flogging top; the master is still the one in charge, he's just having something done to him. The roles of sadist and masochist overlap with other roles, and many people identify with different elements of more than one. Sometimes the overlap is easily recognized, like a submissive masochist bottom who enjoys being flogged to experience both the pain and the submission to his dominant's flogger. But there could also be a sadistic submissive who enjoys piercing masochist bottoms.

Some people take on the role of dominant or submissive expressly for a scene, like top or bottom, and shed that role when the scene ends. For others, being dominant or submissive is not about role playing but is a much bigger part of their identity and relationships. Some dominants can't turn their desire to dominate on and off at will, and they describe dominance as very similar to how people define sexual orientation: these dominants are attracted to and interested in submissives, they see the world through their dominant lens, and their dominance is a constant in their sexual and BDSM interactions.

CHAPTER 4

SEXUAL POWER GAMES:
PLEASURE AND ORGASM CONTROL

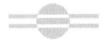

I feel a kind of freedom in consensual objectification and being used as an implement of pleasure or putting my own desires aside in order to serve another individual.

—MADISON

One way to explore dominance and submission is through sexual power games. Sexual power games are role-playing scenarios that use sex as the central tool for control. They often revolve around giving or withholding certain types of stimulation and pleasure, ordering the submissive to perform sex on herself or you, and controlling the submissive's orgasms. Remember that as with other kinky activities, consent is key; so when I use the terms *control*, *order*, *force*, or *torture*, I use them in the context of a scene where people have agreed to consensual dominance and submission.

Tease and Torment

◇◇◇◇◇◇◇

> *Teasing builds tension, anticipation, and arousal.*

Tease and torment is a fun game where the dominant is not only clearly in charge but uses that power to torment the submissive. The idea here is to get your submissive nice and turned on, squirming in pleasure, and then, back off. This is where you stop what you're doing to him, and watch him squirm even more. Put your mouth just an inch away from her pussy and stay there. Turn the vibrator down or off suddenly and don't let her have the controls. Stop fucking her. Hover over her lips just barely touching them. Then, tease. Don't let her get close enough to your hand, mouth, cock, or body to have what she craves. You can combine this game with bondage to make it even more difficult for her to get what she wants. Teasing builds tension, anticipation, and arousal. It puts what your partner desires just out of reach. This can lead to someone asking, begging, pleading, or even bargaining ("I'll give you the best blow job if you just fuck me afterward.") Eventually, you will give in and let her have what she wants, and by then, she'll be so beside herself, the payoff for both of you will be even bigger.

Forced Masturbation

This is a good one to play whether you're in the same room, in separate places, or connecting long distance via phone, instant messenger, text, or Skype. It's easy—the dominant orders the submissive to masturbate. This is a great way to exercise control over her pleasure: she gets to have it, but only when you say so. In fact, maybe she can only touch herself with your permission. Perhaps you give her instructions about exactly how she should do it, and she must follow your directions to the letter or risk punishment. Maybe she needs to describe to you in detail what she's doing, what she's fantasizing about, and what she wants you to do to her. Maybe she needs to get over her shyness and perform for you, give you a show. Maybe she must dedicate her orgasm to you or say your name when she comes, or ask your permission before she has an orgasm. Whatever way you design it, this once solitary activity which was her domain alone now belongs to you.

You can also direct your submissive to masturbate when you're not around. Order her to do it with a specific toy or wearing a particular outfit. Tell her to write up a report of her activities and send it to you. Get creative with your requests; you'll keep her on her toes and you on her mind whenever she masturbates. These can be great homework exercises for couples in long-distance relationships, and they help keep the D/s dynamic present even when you are not physically near each other.

Orgasm Control

◇◇◇◇◇◇◇◇

Imagine if your ability to orgasm was decided by someone else. If you like being at someone's mercy and handing over control of your pleasure, then this kind of surrender may really appeal to you as a submissive. For dominants, do you like to take charge of your partner's body and use sex as a way to control her? *Orgasm control* can take several different forms, each of them a different kind of sexual power play.

One very popular element of dominant/submissive role play is when the dominant requires the submissive to first ask permission in order to have an orgasm. It's a simple, yet deeply symbolic act that says, "I control you. Your orgasms belong to me." Some people write it into their contracts. Basically, the submissive

> *For dominants, do you like to take charge of your partner's body and use sex as a way to control her?*

must always ask the dominant's permission before having an orgasm. Usually, the rule means that as the submissive is right on the edge of coming, he has to pause, ask (or beg), and the dominant can decide to extend or deny permission for him to have an orgasm. Creative dominants can require a task first ("Lick my boots!") or administer ten strokes of the paddle before permission is given. Orgasm control is a ritual that not only reinforces the dominant/submissive dynamic but is also such a fun power game to play!

Speaking of denying permission, *orgasm denial* is another form of control—one that's a bit more devious (and, yes, even sadistic). When the submissive asks for permission, your answer is confident and resounding: "No." You can do it as a correction, punishment, or just to see the look on her face. Denying orgasm makes a submissive squirm, squeal, beg, plead, all while getting more turned on in the process. It's a great way to take someone to the edge of climax, then flip the switch. You get bonus points for incorporating sex toys into this game, like vibrators, Kegel balls (also called Ben Wa balls), dildos, or butt plugs—since they'll make it even more difficult for her to not come.

It's another kind of tease and torment sure to drive her crazy, where the reward—a much-anticipated orgasm *when you say so*—is even sweeter. Or perhaps the reward is delayed, a few hours or a few days.

On the other end of the spectrum is the *forced orgasm*. Let me start with a disclaimer: if your partner has trouble achieving orgasm, this is not the game to play. It could create tension, anxiety, shame, and fear, and that's not what we're after at all. But if your partner is reliably orgasmic, then this is another fun way to control her. Think of it as making your partner have an orgasm on demand. When you feel like she's getting close (or she has told you she is, as instructed), you can demand that she come. Or you can put her in some nice bondage, then strap a vibrator to her clitoris, so she has no choice but to come. The dominant gets to call the shots, the submissive gets to follow the command and come: win-win!

Sexual Service

◇◇◇◇◇◇

Dominants can require all kinds of service from submissives, but sexual service is one of the most popular fantasies people have. Demanding sexual service and making your pleasure his *only* priority is a clear way to exert power over a submissive. Not only can you make a specific demand, but

> *Providing sexual service is a big turn-on for many submissives.*

you can enhance the experience in different ways: require that he be sexually available to you whenever you want; provide specific directions about how you want something done to you; make the task more difficult by binding his hands so he can only use his mouth; put a hood on him and tell him you're going to use his body for your pleasure; or combine service for you that turns him on, like cunnilingus, with orgasm denial for him.

Providing sexual service is a big turn-on for many submissives who enjoy being focused on the dominant's pleasure and/or being sexually used or objectified. Some really enjoy the role of the sexually available, willing, and able sex slave who could be called on at a moment's notice (provided it works with everyone's hectic schedule, of course). They enjoy creating a "non-negotiable" sex scenario (which, of course, they've actually negotiated beforehand): there is no question about who initiates, who does what, or what's expected. They don't have to overthink anything, just do what they are told. For some, this allows them the freedom and permission to be constantly horny, ready to go, even "oversexed," since that is part of being a good sex slave.

CHAPTER 5

SENSORY DEPRIVATION:
BLINDFOLDS, HOODS, AND EARPLUGS

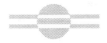

I'm blindfolded and gagged on a pillow in a cold basement. I can feel the cool air and hear water dripping. I hear high heels coming closer and am struck across my ass and chest, slowly increasing in intensity. She straddles my shoulders after a good flogging and orders me to pleasure her. Right before she is about to come, she moves away and finishes herself off while all I can do is listen to her moans and screams.

—CHASE

When you take away someone's sense of sight or sound, their other senses become heightened. When you're blindfolded, noises sound louder, smells are more intense, and even the lightest touch can send chills down the spine. When you can't hear anything or you can hear only one particular sound, you focus on what you can feel, smell, possibly see (if you can), or simply sense around you. *Sensory deprivation play* focuses on depriving someone of sight or sound—with blindfolds, hoods, earplugs, headphones, or some combination of these. This deprivation can help to put someone in a particular frame of mind; people wearing these devices often feel curious and excited as they anticipate what might come next in a scene. Sensory deprivation toys can also help someone focus on what's happening to their body, making each sensation stronger.

Blindfolds

Blindfolds come in polyester, satin, leather, and other fabrics, and it's a matter of personal taste which you prefer. Some sleep masks—those that really block out light—work very well as blindfolds. Some blindfolds have an elastic strap; others fasten with Velcro or a buckle. An adjustable elastic strap is preferable to one that isn't adjustable, although if there is enough give, a nonadjustable blindfold should be fine; just make sure the blindfold fits snugly but is not too tight. If you're going to be lying on your back most of the time, then you may not want a blindfold with a buckle, since it can become uncomfortable against the back of your head pretty quickly. If you want to obscure someone's vision but not take away their sight entirely, try a sheer scarf that's folded several times.

Putting a blindfold on someone is a great way to neutralize the environment around them. If they can't see, suddenly they have to rely on you to tell them what's going on—or not; this is a great opportunity to shift a bottom's sense of reality, spin a fantasy, or control what they know (or think they know). For some bottoms, a blindfold immediately makes them feel submissive; for others, it puts them off balance enough that they can slip more easily into a fantasy. Blindfolds can also give beginner tops a boost of confidence—it's easier to project a sense of confidence, discipline, and precision if your bottom can't see you fumble with a flogger!

People who wear contact lenses and a blindfold for a long period of time may find that their lenses dry out or become uncomfortable; keep lens drops handy or have submissives take their lenses out before you begin. When a blindfold comes off, the person will usually be disoriented and extra sensitive to light, so give them some time to readjust to being able to see again.

> *Blindfolds can also give beginner tops a boost of confidence.*

Hoods

◇◇◇◇◇◇◇◇

If you enjoy the sense of helplessness that blindfolds provide, wearing a hood will take it to another level. Hoods can be made of different kinds of material from spandex to leather, but they have one thing in common: breathability. That may mean small holes in fabric, perforations in leather, or eye/nose/

mouth cutouts. Like blindfolds, hoods obscure your vision, but they can do something more; some people have a profound loss of identity when they wear a hood. They can immediately feel small and submissive. Think about it: when your face is completely covered, you can feel erased, dehumanized, or objectified. This can be a useful tool if, for example, a bottom enjoys being "used" as a sex slave; a hood can transform someone into simply a mouth available to please her master whenever he chooses. It's common to combine sensory deprivation with bondage (which I'll discuss about in Chapters 7 and 8).

Earplugs and Headphones

Our sense of sound is one important way that we process information about what's happening around us. Like a blindfold, taking away someone's ability to hear can heighten their other senses and help them to focus on exactly what you want them to: the feel of ice melting and dripping between their breasts, the pinch of a clamp around their nipple, the sting of a cane. Using earplugs (available in most drugstores), you not only alter what a bottom hears but also turn up the volume of their own breathing, which can be an intense experience that connects them to their body and what's happening to it.

Another way to play with the sense of sound is to control *what* the bottom hears. This isn't exactly sensory deprivation; it's more like sensory manipulation. Think about walking into an empty room. You hear a heavy metal song. Or a piano concerto. Or the deep bass of techno music. Each one conveys a different tone. Put a pair of headphones on a bottom to fill their ears with a desired soundtrack, and it can set the mood for your scene. Perhaps the fantasy is to be taken advantage of under the bleachers during a football game. A soundtrack of cheerleading chants can help bring that to life. Or you want her to imagine having sex in public at an orgy. Put on your favorite group-sex scene in a porn movie, and you've got the sounds of other people having sex and coming all around you.

CHAPTER 6

SENSATION PLAY:
MASSAGE OIL CANDLES, NIPPLE CLAMPS, AND MORE

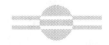

Gentle. Ticklish. Hot. Cold. Rough. Soft. Smooth. For many people, kink is about experiencing lots of different, sometimes intense, sensations that go far beyond just genital stimulation. I discussed sensory deprivation in the previous chapter, but now it's time to ramp up all the senses, especially touch: this chapter is about sensory *stimulation* that focuses on creating unique sensations on the skin. Sensation play approaches the flesh of the body like a sculptor begins with a fresh lump of clay—her body is a blank canvas to manipulate and stimulate with different textures, temperatures, and "torture."

Feathers

◇◇◇◇◇◇◇

There's a reason that in the popular French maid fantasy, the maid is usually carrying a feather duster, and it doesn't have anything to do with cleaning the house! Feathers are sensual, luxurious tools that feel great against the skin and stimulate our touch receptors. They can stroke, flutter, tickle, and tease the flesh. They are a fun way to get someone in the mood without intimidating them, so they are a good bet for beginners and lovers who aren't ready just yet to bring out the whip.

Combining a feather with a blindfold or bondage can make your partner feel like they are at your mercy. You can buy a large single feather (like a giant ostrich feather) or a feather tickler made of many feathers attached to a handle (similar to a duster). Run a feather tickler down the entire length of your partner's body. Brush the feathers lightly against the skin, then follow each swipe

> *Feathers are sensual, luxurious tools that feel great against the skin and stimulate our touch receptors.*

with a kiss. If you're feeling playful, you can use your feather to torture him as you target his ticklish spots. If tickling turns both of you on, then go for it.

Edible Body Paint and Dust

If you love the idea of licking chocolate sauce, whipped cream, honey, and other goodies off your partner's body, then you'll love edible body paint and dust. Imagine soft baby powder sprinkled on your skin, then nibbled off by someone you love. You can experience that sensation with edible body dust. Some dusts come with a feather, so you can combine the sensuality of feathers against the skin with a delicious powder. Edible body paints are just as tasty as sundae toppings, but these paints are safe for the body, moisturizing to the skin, and easy to clean up afterward. Edible body paints come in different colors and flavors and offer all sorts of fun opportunities. Create a colorful masterpiece on your naked body. Draw a bikini on and have him take it off. Write naughty words on your body and ask your partner to lick them off. Paint your partner's sensitive spots, then erase them with your mouth.

Massage Oil Candles

Candles are a wonderful way to set a romantic mood, and many couples light them to create some sexy ambiance in the bedroom. Some folks fantasize about another use for those candles: they want to seductively drip hot wax all over their partner's body or have it drizzled on themselves. It looks great in the movies, but the reality doesn't always live up to the hype: if you use the wrong kind of candle, the wax can actually burn someone's skin. Even if you get a candle with a low burn temperature, you're still left with a lot of cooled wax to clean up. Massage candles not only address and fix these common issues, but they combine two activities with one product. They burn at a very low temperature, making it gentle and safe to use without fear of hurting your partner by scorching their skin. Light

> *A sensual massage is a great way to start an evening of sexy fun.*

the candle and let the wax begin to melt. Lift your hand up and away from your partner's body (the farther away the candle, the cooler the wax will be when it hits the skin). Once you've drizzled your partner's body with warm wax, start rubbing your fingers into it, and it will transform into silky smooth massage oil. Now you're ready to give an erotic massage! A sensual massage is a great way to start an evening of sexy fun. You don't need to be a licensed masseuse to give a good massage; you just need to be generous, listen to your partner, and use the healing power of touch.

You can drip hot wax almost anywhere on the body except the face and genitals. The most important thing to keep in mind with massage oil is that it does in fact contain oil, so it can stain sheets, fabric, and clothes and may be hard to clean up; make sure you put a towel down first. Oil-based products should not get near your genitals if you're planning to have sex. Oil-based products are bad for vaginas and can cause vaginal infections.

You can follow up these warm sensations with an ice cube to surprise your partner, shift the temperature of the skin, or cool things down.

Stimulating Gels and Creams

We all know that genitals are very sensitive, but some folks like to make them even more so. Stimulating gels and creams like Rocket Balm, Flower Balm, and Please Pleasure Cream do just that. I recommend the products that contain some kind of natural stimulant, like menthol or peppermint, over those with chemical stimulants or numbing agents. Stimulating gels and creams created for men can be used to stimulate the head and frenulum of the penis; apply a small amount, and in a few seconds, the area will start to tingle. Those made for women can be used on the clitoris and are formulated to boost the arousal process and make her more sensitive. When you put a tiny bit on the hood or the underside of the clitoris, the area tingles, blood rushes to the genitals, and the entire vulva gets swollen and aroused. I don't recommend you put them on other parts of the labia, and they should definitely not be used internally. You can also use them on men or women's nipples for extra sensation.

Blind Sensation

* * * * *

A blindfold can be added to the mix with any of the activities in this chapter, which will build anticipation, amplify the sensation, and keep your partner guessing. Once she's blindfolded, use a bunch of different things to drag across the skin. Think wooden chopsticks, fur or another very soft material, ice cubes, your hand in a leather glove, or your nails (if your partner likes being scratched). Remember without sight, something like a simple butter knife will feel like a sharp knife but won't mark or cut the skin.

Nipple Clamps

Chests, breasts, and nipples are all wonderful erogenous zones on our bodies. Both men's and women's nipples can be very sensitive, though the level of sensitivity varies from person to person. Lots of folks like their nipples licked, sucked, rolled between fingers, and tugged gently. If you like your nipples twisted, tweaked, and, especially, pinched during sex, then you may like nipple clamps.

Nipple clamps are small clips attached to a chain, and they come in a wide variety of styles. The best starter set for beginners are tweezer-style or adjustable nipple clamps. Other nipple clamps, as well as similar pinching implements (like clothes-pins, paper clips, or hair clips) are not adjustable at all; their clamping strength might be too intense to start out with for a lot of people. Tweezer-style nipple clamps have a small ring that lets you adjust how much they clamp.

With adjustable clamps, you can start out with the loosest clamping and work your way up to a tighter and more severe pinch. Take your partner's nipple and rub it until it's hard. Place each side of the clamp on the nipple, then slowly begin to slide the ring toward the nipple to tighten it. Check in with your partner to see what feels good. When you put a clamp on a part of the body, you cut off the circulation to that area. The nipples can get very sensitive, so tugging on the chain between the clamps sends a zing throughout the body. While it hurts to varying degrees when you put the clamps on and tug at them, it feels a hell of a lot worse when the clamps come off. The blood quickly rushes back to the area in a big burst, and bang, your brain registers pain. So, if your partner is a beginner, leave nipple clamps on for less than a minute before you take them off. You can gradually work your way up to longer amounts of time, but you shouldn't leave clamps on for more than fifteen minutes.

> *Check in with your partner to see what feels good.*

CHAPTER 7

BONDAGE:
BASICS AND DIY

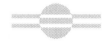

Bondage Basics

When many people recall their first experience of bondage, it usually reaches all the way back to childhood. As part of cops-and-robbers or similar kids' games, someone had to be restrained at some point. You'd grab a necktie, belt, scarf, or something else from one of your parents' closets and tie up the bad guys. Some people look back on those experiences as fun memories. Bondage enthusiasts usually remember the first time they were tied up (or tied someone else up) with a lot more detail and glee.

For grown-ups, bondage is an erotic activity with endless possibilities. If you've ever held down your lover's hands while you

> *And being restrained is a way to submit, surrender, and give oneself over to another.*

were having sex or pinned a partner down to the bed with your body, then you've practiced a form of bondage.

Bondage is incredibly versatile and can cover lots of erotic territory, from teasing to torment, and everything in between. It's an ideal vehicle to explore power dynamics, since restraining someone embodies dominance, control, power, and authority. And being restrained is a way to submit, surrender, and give oneself over to another.

There are some basic rules for bondage that apply to anything you use to restrain someone or bind a part of their body. Whether it's Velcro, a belt with a buckle, or a knot, you should always make sure whatever you put someone in is safe. First, always have a pair of safety scissors nearby, in case you have to get someone out of bondage very quickly. Safety scissors have a blunt-edged blade to prevent injury when the scissors are held against skin. They're available in most drugstores.

Whether you tie them in bows or fancy knots, cuffs around the ankles and wrist should be snug but not too tight; you should be able to put two fingers between the item and the person's skin. You never want bondage to put too much strain on parts of the body; the person won't be able to be in that bondage for very long. Better to make your captive more comfortable, so she or he can stay tied up for as long as you want! You should also check in periodically with your partner to make sure that everything still feels okay. If the person in bondage feels pain, tingling, or numbness, take the restraint off immediately.

DIY Bondage

There are many different types of bondage toys; this chapter will cover those you can make yourself— common household items you can repurpose for bondage. The next chapter will cover items you can buy at a sex toy or fetish store, including collars, bondage tape, wrist and ankle cuffs, and bondage tether kits.

One of the bonuses of bondage is that you can do it without any fancy equipment and use what's nearby. First, let me tell you what *not* to use. Athletic tape and duct tape—really sticky tape of any kind—can be too sticky and bind to the skin; if left on long enough, it can be difficult to get off without taking some skin with it, like the worst Band-Aid removal ever. Also, you may have some plastic zip ties in your toolbox, but just leave them there. Zip ties can close too tightly and cut off circulation, plus the hard plastic can abrade the thin skin around your wrists. Although you might think it looks cool, avoid metal chain of any kind; like the zip ties, metal against delicate skin is a recipe for sore wrists.

Neckties, silk (or silky) scarves, and bathrobe ties are all much better choices. They are a good length for wrist and ankle bondage, and they're soft, so they won't cut or irritate the skin. First, put the bottom in the position you'd ultimately like to have her stay in; if you want her hands above her head, for instance, put them there. To bind the wrists, have the bottom put her hands together, palms facing each other. Slide the tie or scarf under her wrists. You can bring the two ends together or double them around if there is enough length. Simply finish with a bow or regular knot.

One sexy idea is to arrive for a date without any gear at all, slowly strip down, and use what you're wearing to tie up your lover. Things like suspenders, pantyhose, and stockings all make great bondage materials. Because these items are stretchy, it's very important not to bind them too tightly. Since the material has give to it, it's a good choice for bottoms who like to move around a lot, and it's good for beginners who want to know they could "break out" of it fairly easily if they need to.

If you and your partner are interested in moving beyond just wrists and ankles, athletic wrap (like an

> *One sexy idea is to arrive for a date without any gear at all.*

Ace bandage) offers you more to work with. If you want to bind someone's arms to their sides so they truly cannot move them, these inexpensive rolls of stretchy material can cover a lot of surface area. Remember not to stretch it too tightly, just tight enough to hold. When you get to the end of the roll, you can use the metal clips or a piece of masking or athletic tape.

CHAPTER 8

MORE BONDAGE:
RESTRAINTS, BONDAGE TAPE, GAGS, AND COLLARS

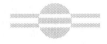

The most common image associated with bondage and sex is a pair of shiny metal handcuffs. I see them in people's bedrooms, they're sold at some sex shops, and they make a frequent appearance in erotica, but they really are not safe to use to restrain someone. Most handcuffs do not have a working safety latch to keep them from closing too tightly around the wrist; they can cut off your circulation, cut into your wrists, and do serious damage to someone. And let's not even discuss how many people have lost the key to their handcuffs—what an unfortunate mishap to explain! If you find fabric- or faux-fur-covered handcuffs, still be wary; they can be very uncomfortable and equally unsafe. The only time you should use a pair of covered handcuffs is if there is padding between the fabric and the metal and there's a safety latch to keep them from closing too tightly. Even with those features, there is still the pesky key issue!

If you're ready to invest in some bondage gear, you will find lots of choices at a good reputable sex toy store. In this chapter, I'll discuss some of the most popular, including bondage tape, wrist and ankle cuffs, collars, leashes, gags, and bondage kits.

Bondage Tape

Have you ever seen a movie where someone gets tied up with duct tape? It's quick, easy, and good guys and bad guys alike always seem to have it handy. Duct tape is great for lots of things, but in the real world, bondage is not one of them. Luckily, some pervy people have invented an alternative!

Bondage tape is made of a thin plastic, comes

> *Some practice isn't a bad idea.*

in several colors, and is available at most sex toy stores. It comes in a two-inch-wide roll that looks a lot like packing tape, but this tape isn't sticky, so it's safe for your skin. Bondage tape clings to itself, which is how it stays in place, but it won't stick to hair or skin. I love bondage tape because it's inexpensive and easy to use—you don't even have to know how to tie a knot to tie someone up. Some practice isn't a bad idea, though; ideally you want to keep it as flat against the skin as possible, since when it bunches up, it can cause pinching. Wrap it around wrists, arms, thighs, and ankles; make a blindfold; tie someone to a chair. When you're ready to set your captive free, you can unroll it (which takes some patience) and reuse it, or simply cut it off and throw it away.

If you like bondage tape, there is a DIY (although admittedly more cumbersome) version: ordinary plastic wrap, which is probably in your kitchen right now! Plastic wrap can do many of the same things that bondage tape does, except it's actually stickier, so it can be more awkward to use, and it's not reusable. Keep those safety scissors handy to cut it off!

Wrist and Ankle Cuffs

◇◇◇◇◇◇◇

Wrist and ankle cuffs come in a variety of price ranges and styles and can be made of nylon, vinyl, leather, rubber, or

> *Cuffs should not be too loose, but they should never be tight.*

other materials. If they are not made of a soft material, consider getting cuffs that are lined with some cushioning, like fleece, to make them more comfortable (which means you or your partner can stay in them longer!). Wrap wrist cuffs just above the wrist bone (away from the hand) and secure them; they usually have Velcro or buckles. Cuffs should not be too loose, but they should never be tight. You can use wrist cuffs alone, ankle cuffs, or both.

Once the cuffs are on, you have some choices to further restrain your partner. Each cuff has a ring on it to attach things to, and you can use a snap hook or carabiner (found at hardware stores) or other type of clip to attach the cuffs to each other. You can clip cuffs together over someone's head, in front of them, or behind them. The important thing is that the position you "lock" their arms into isn't putting too much strain on their body. Or you may not want their wrists together, but spread apart, and tethered to something sturdy. This is especially true of ankles, since most people prefer to have their partner's legs spread for easy access. Slip a long scarf, a belt, or a piece of rope through the ring and tie each wrist or ankle to a chair, the slats in your headboard, the bedposts, or something else solid and stable. If you don't have a bed that you can tie someone to, check out the bondage kits described below.

Collars and Leashes

While they've become more mainstream and some people wear them as a fashion statement, I'm old school when it comes to collars. To me, a collar is both a form of bondage and a symbol. It may signify ownership, submission, subservience, surrender, and a whole range of other power dynamics. For many, when a lover puts a collar around their neck, it helps them to give up control and become more submissive. Putting a collar on someone is also a great way to begin a role-playing scene, to transition from your real-life personalities into dominant and submissive, master and slave, or whatever roles you've chosen for the scene. Like other bondage toys, collars can be made of leather, rubber, nylon, and other materials; some collars have Velcro or buckles, and others have a ring where you can insert a lock. For the fashion conscious among you—you know who you are—you can often get a collar to match your wrist and ankle restraints. A collar should be snug around the neck, but never tight, choking, or cutting off circulation; make sure you can fit two fingers between the collar and the person's neck. You can grab the front ring of a collar to pull someone toward you, but never yank someone's collar or drag them by the neck.

Leashes often go with collars in other contexts, and so it is with kink, where they can be a nice addition to a collar. You can lead someone around the room on a collar and leash to demonstrate their submission to you. This is something you don't do ordinarily, so it's one way to begin a scene that can get both partners in the right frame of mind. Using a leash is meant to be playful; you can give a gentle tug to remind her who's boss or lead her to where you want to fuck her. While it may be tempting, you never want to pull someone by the leash or jerk the leash suddenly with any force—no whiplash injuries, please!

Mouth Gags

Similar to taking away a person's sight or hearing with sensory deprivation, taking away someone's ability to speak can have a variety of effects. Since talking is the number one way we express ourselves and exchange information, it's something we often take for granted and do without thinking. Making it impossible for a bottom to use spoken language to communicate can be a way to establish your dominance and exercise control over them. Think of a mouth gag as bondage for their mouth—you can hold their voice captive! You can create a system of hand signals and other physical cues to communicate. Rendering a chatty bottom speechless is often a sight to behold: she can become frustrated, focused, submissive, or some combination. Either way, it's a dramatic shift that a dominant can use to his advantage. Another thing happens when you wear a gag for a while: you drool. It cannot be avoided, but it can be humiliating and embarrassing for those bottoms who enjoy those feelings in an erotic context. A ball gag can also quiet them from screaming so the neighbors don't call the cops!

> *Think of a mouth gag as bondage for their mouth.*

A mouth gag usually has two parts: the part that sits in the mouth and a strap attached to either side of it that you can fasten around the head to keep it in. You want to find a gag that is comfortable enough to wear for a little while and doesn't put strain on the mouth and jaw. Although you will find lots of hard plastic ball gags, I prefer something with a little give to it. So look for a rubber or silicone ball with some flexibility. A gag that's too big will make a bottom feel like they're choking, which isn't any fun. There are other types of gags as well: gags that are similar to a ball gag, but come in a different shape, like a dog bone, a penis, or a horse bit; gags with a ring that holds the mouth open; and inflatable mouth gags. You can also create your own gag with a bandanna tied around a bottom's mouth or a balled-up pair of underwear. Be creative, improvise, but always make sure your bottom can breathe easily and his jaw isn't under pressure.

Whenever you use a gag, your bottom needs to have a safe signal (or signals) to replace her safeword(s). Use something out of the ordinary, like stomping her foot or holding something in her hand that she can drop.

Bondage Kits

Bondage kits come complete with several different pieces that work together to create a great bondage experience. Some kits make it possible to do bondage in an ordinary bedroom without any fancy equipment; if you don't have a slatted headboard or a four-poster bed, you can transform any ordinary bed into your own bondage playground! Here are some of the best kits available:

Sportsheets Under the Bed Restraint System: This clever kit is perfect for folks who want to be able to tie someone down to the bed but don't have the type of bed that you can attach anything to. Two long, strong nylon straps go between the mattress and the box spring or around the bedframe, and they can be adjusted to fit any size bed. Lay them vertically and the straps come around the head and foot of the bed, resting at the top and bottom of the mattress so you can restrain hands and feet there. Lay them horizontally and restrain someone's arms and legs on either side of the bed. At both ends of each strap is a clip that you attach the nylon and Velcro cuffs to (all are included in the kit). Of course, you can use any set of wrist and ankle cuffs with the straps.

The Sportsheet Bondage Bed Sheet Set: Available in queen and king size, the Sportsheet is a velvety mattress cover. It comes with four "anchor pads," thick pads with Velcro that stick to the sheet and stay in place; each pad has a clip on it to which you can attach wrist and ankle cuffs. Once your sweetie is clipped to the pads, he isn't going anywhere!

Liberator Shapes Black Label: Liberator Shapes are firm pillow-like shapes that help you create different (and

> *Once your sweetie is clipped to the pads, he isn't going anywhere!*

supported) angles of the body during sex. The company makes a line of shapes which feature black velvety covers that come equipped with easy-to-use bondage attachments to which you can clip cuffs with a special quick-release clip (also made by Liberator Shapes).

Sportsheets Deluxe Door Jam Kit: Have you ever fantasized about being able to tie up your partner in a standing position, but you're not quite ready to invest in an expensive wooden frame, or you can't drill holes for eye hooks into the molding? You can turn any doorway into a bondage device with this inventive kit. Slip these four nylon straps with clips on one end and plastic stoppers on the other over the top of the door and under the bottom. Close the door, and voila, you've got a sturdy, nonpermanent bondage setup right in your house! These are also great for romantic getaways, since they won't cause any damage to a hotel room.

CHAPTER 9

SMACK!
SPANKING, PADDLES, AND CROPS

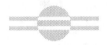

Lots of people love a good spanking. Don't just take my word for it: there are hundreds of adult movies devoted to spanking, dozens of erotic websites, and over the years, there has been more than one magazine devoted to the subject. For some, spanking goes along with fantasy role playing—naughty schoolgirls and unruly boys disciplined at the hands of a cruel teacher, a stern governess, or an unforgiving nun. Perhaps the play is closer to home, with Mommy or Daddy wielding the unrelenting hairbrush. Others use spanking as a tool of dominance and submission, an expression of control, humiliation, and punishment (or reward!). A spanking can be just a spanking, but decide in advance what the spanking will mean in the context of your play. Many pervy people report that spanking was the first kinky thing they did.

It can be dreaded and scary or sweet and sexy, but it is undeniably a very intimate act. Get your bottom in a comfortable position: lying over your lap, on all fours, or bent over the bed, a stool, or a table. Like most things, it's best to start out slowly, beginning with light, gentle taps before moving on to full-handed slaps. Not only does this make the spanking more fun, but the bottom can usually take it longer and harder if you warm up the ass first. Begin alternating

> *Many pervy people report that spanking was the first kinky thing they did.*

sides with a light spank, followed by a massage. Keep your hand as close to the ass as possible in the beginning; the farther away you take your hand, the less control you have over hitting the exact spot you are aiming for and the more likely you are to hit it too hard. Remember, the more aroused she is, the more enjoyable the spanking will be for both of you, so don't hold back on stroking the other nearby parts, too!

As you move on to harder slaps, experiment with different sensations—the tips of your fingers versus your entire hand, the middle of the ass versus right where the cheek curves into the thigh. Add variety to your spanks by wearing a pair of soft leather gloves (for a different sensation), wetting your hand (for a stingier slap), or place your hand on a heating pad first (for a warm spank).

Many people get very turned on by spanking. Slapping someone's butt cheeks can be gentle and sensual or deliberate and painful; either way, the consistent smacks release endorphins into the bloodstream and fuel the body's arousal. While the ass is usually the target of a spanking, you can also slap the butt cheeks, thighs, and other fleshy parts of the body; always avoid bones and joints, such as the tailbone and the back of the knees, and organs like the kidneys. All these rules apply if you use your hand or one of the toys discussed next.

To add a little something more to a spanking,

position a vibrator between her legs so it's nestled against her clit exactly where she likes it. A wand-style clitoral vibrator with a large head, or a rounded one meant for her to rub against work really well for this. With each spank, her body will press into the vibrator with a little more pressure and the vibration will feel more intense. Or slip a set of Ben Wa balls (also called "Kegel balls" or "smart balls") inside her. As you spank her butt cheeks, the balls will move against each other inside her, which will create a different kind of vibrating sensation. If she's on her stomach or leaned over something, gravity will work in her favor, and the balls can actually massage her G-spot. Have her clench her pelvic muscles around the balls to intensify the sensation. You could also use an insertable vibrator or a dildo to combine penetration with a rhythmic spanking. As the spanking progresses, the toy will move inside her (or you can move it for her), delivering double the pleasure.

You can also spank or slap the genitals, but start out very gently. The tissue of the vulva and penis are much less fleshy than other parts and a lot more sensitive. To spank a vulva, put your hand up, fingers together facing the vulva. Start with light taps, and see how she responds. For some women, this will simply be too intense, but for others, especially once they are aroused, it can be both exciting and stimulating. Try concentrating on the pubic mound and above the clitoral hood; or, spank over the hood directly. In between slaps and taps, use your fingers to stroke her labia and clitoris. Talk to her, pay attention to her body language, and only escalate your spanks when you know she's enjoying it. To spank a penis, hold the shaft with one hand and slap with the other. Try light taps on the head and see how he responds. You can increase the speed and strength of the slaps if he's into it.

Paddles, Slappers, and Crops

You'd be surprised at just how much impact you can have with your own bare hand, but using toys for spanking and slapping is lots of fun, too.

As a general rule, when spanking or slapping

someone with a toy, you want to concentrate on fleshy areas of the body like the ass cheeks, the back of the thighs, the inner thighs, and the back. The chest can also be slapped as well as the breasts, but extra care should be taken with the breasts—don't use anything too heavy. And again, always avoid bones, joints, and organs (be especially careful of the tailbone and the kidneys when slapping someone's back or butt).

Look no further than your own house for some great DIY spanking toys—like wooden spoons, spatulas, hairbrushes, or rulers. All of these tools provide different materials and different sensation possibilities. Make sure you try out a DIY toy on yourself to get a sense of what kind of smack it produces, how much force you need to use, and what it feels like.

You can purchase a range of spanking toys— like paddles, slappers, and crops—at sex toy and BDSM stores and websites. Most of these tools can produce a

> *Look no further than your own house for some great DIY spanking toys.*

light sensation or a heavy, painful one depending on how much force is behind it.

Most paddles have a broad round or oval striking part and a short handle. Paddles are made of leather, vinyl, rubber, wood, acrylic, and other materials—generally the harder the material, the more intense the sensation it can produce. They come in a variety of colors, and some feature one side made of leather or wood and the other side covered in faux (or real) fur. This double-sided paddle is delightful, since you have both soft and hard in one toy. You can begin with strokes of fur, move on to taps, slaps, and smacks of leather, then alternate between the two. A firm slap of leather against the flesh followed by the soothing rub of sensual fur feels amazing. Some paddles feature stars, hearts, or other shapes on them. The idea behind these is that the better you get with your aim and the more consistent your smacks are, the more likely the shape will create an imprint in your bottom's butt cheeks (or elsewhere). This way, they can have an artistic reminder of the spanking.

Crops are long rods with a small flat loop or a

> **Crops are great for beginners who are just starting to explore spanking and slapping.**

solid piece of leather on the end. The end piece is the part you slap with, which means that of paddles, slappers, and crops, crops have the smallest slapping area. Because of their design, crops can be used more effectively on smaller areas that a paddle may be too big for—like breasts, nipples, vulvas, or the place where the inner thigh meets the pubic area. As with other tools, start out slowly with light taps, and increase the intensity as your partner responds. Crops are great for beginners who are just starting to explore spanking and slapping because you can experiment with the sensations without doing very much damage.

Slappers tend to be longer than paddles and rectangular, and have a more narrow spanking area. A slapper can be made of one single piece of leather, one piece cut into several strips, or two pieces of leather sewn together at one end. Slappers with multiple pieces of leather tend to make a much louder noise than paddles, so they can be as much a sensory head trip as a physical one. In general, slappers can produce a harder slap or a stingier one compared to a paddle, which has a larger surface area to diffuse the impact. If you've enjoyed hand spanking, but crave something more intense or with more of a "bite," a slapper may be a good fit for you.

Before you introduce your sweetheart to it, it's a good idea for you to try out a paddle, slapper, or crop on a fleshy part of your own body to get an idea of what your partner is going to feel. The key to a good spanking with a paddle, slapper, or crop is to start slowly, warm up the area, and not rush to spank too hard. Begin with very light flicks, and alternate each one with a nice rub of your hand. You want to gradually build up to firmer swats. Talk to your partner, pay attention to body language, and pace the spanking accordingly.

I like to alternate the sting of a smack with a warm and fuzzy feeling, like the rub of a fur mitt or the tickle of a feather. To create a combination of hot and cold, after a particularly hard spanking or in between two mild sets, rub an ice cube over the skin.

CHAPTER 10

SMACK HARDER:
FLOGGERS AND CANES

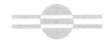

Floggers

Floggers—sometimes called cat-o'-nine-tails or simply whips—have a handle and multiple "tails"—strips of material which are the same length and width. Inexpensive, light floggers (sometimes called "fantasy floggers") can be found in many sex toy stores and are good for beginners or those interested in exploring light flogging. If you're looking for a starter flogger, I recommend one that is relatively short, since it's easier to control. If you want leather, make sure the tails are made of a very soft

leather, like deerskin
or suede. Sportsheets
makes floggers with
very thin stretchy pieces

> *You want the right tool for the job.*

of rubber, in several different lengths, which are
good for novices.

Expensive, hand-crafted floggers geared for
kinky people with more experience and skill are
sold at sex and leather shops and BDSM events.
These floggers have handles most often made of
leather, plastic, or wood. The tails (anywhere from
about twenty to fifty) can be made of a variety of
materials, usually different animal hides or rubber.
Well-crafted floggers are beautiful and come in
magnificent colors and designs, but don't make
the mistake of selecting a flogger just because it
looks pretty. You want the right tool for the job.
For example, suede and deerskin floggers produce
a sensual, warm, light thud and are good for beginners. Cowhide floggers are versatile, and they can
create a soft to medium sensation with a tiny bite.
Elk is thicker than deer, and an elkskin flogger
creates a heavy, deep, penetrating thud, so it's better

for experienced floggers; elk is also less common and harder to find. The leather of a bullhide flogger has more density, is much heavier, and has quite a bite. Whips with leather braided tails, or tails with knotted ends are among the most severe and are recommended for experienced players only.

When the tails of a flogger hit the flesh, it can create a range of sensations from light smacks to heavy thuds, depending on the type of flogger and the power behind the strike. Some people enjoy the different sensations a flogger can produce: slaps, stings, and thuds can feel good and release endorphins. If, for example, you very lightly throw a suede flogger, it can feel like a flutter against the skin; put some more power behind it and it can feel like a more solid smack.

It is important for you to learn how to flog someone properly before you incorporate it into a scene. I absolutely recommend that you go to a workshop on flogging or ask an experienced player to give you a personal tutorial. Local BDSM organizations and stores often sponsor workshops by some of the leading practitioners and teachers in the

BDSM community. While you are still getting a grip, so to speak, on flogging, it's a good idea to practice your aim, timing, and technique on an inanimate object like a pillow or a large stuffed animal.

To use a flogger you want to hold the handle and aim the ends of the tails at your "target." You can swing the flogger over your shoulder, then forward to the person's body, or you can swing it sideways (some people refer to the swing as "throwing" the flogger). Start gently and work your way up to more intensity. Like anything else new, it takes lots of practice before you can master it. When I started flogging bottoms, I often put a towel around their necks to protect them from my novice aim which often went off course. It's crucial that a flogging be well-paced, with plenty of warm-up, building up to more and more intensity. Just like spanking and slapping, you should only flog the fleshy parts of the body, like butt cheeks, thighs, and the upper back; always avoid joints, organs, and bones, including the spine, the lower back (because of the kidneys), knees, shins, ankles, elbows, shoulder blades, stomach, head, neck, and face. You can flog the genitals but use a short, gentle flogger and start out very slowly.

Canes

◇◇◇◇◇◇◇◇

In the kink world, a cane is not a long hooked stick that people walk with, but an old-fashioned, long, thin rod, often thought of as an English disciplinary tool. Canes can be made of rattan, acrylic, hard plastic, and other materials. Don't be fooled by their thin, seemingly innocuous appearance; canes can be one of the meanest toys in a dominant's arsenal. These tools may look innocent, but canes can actually really hurt, very easily mark the skin, and even draw blood.

Like spanking, you should only hit someone with a cane on fleshy parts of the body—usually the butt cheeks and thighs—and avoid the kidneys, bones, and joints. You do not need a lot of strength to wield a cane, and a few strokes can leave some nasty marks. The firm stroke of a cane creates a very different sensation than paddles, hands, or floggers:

it is a sharp, biting, burning sensation that spreads from the site of the smack and beyond. Canes are not for the faint-hearted and are definitely an acquired taste.

CHAPTER 11

ROUGH SEX

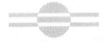

I adore face slapping and hair pulling (as long as they are done properly), and spitting on my pussy or ass as part of my sex play. Throw me down on the bed, or shove me against a wall, and I melt.

—KYLIE

A pink handprint on a pale ass cheek. A fistful of hair. A string of gooey spit dripping down your chin. Nails dragged across flesh. A slap across the face. An order barked with cool confidence. A guttural groan or a high-pitched squeal. These are some of the sights and sounds of rough sex. Although it is obviously intensely physical, there are also strong psychological elements in rough sex. Rough sex tops get turned on by taking control of a partner's body, using physical force, and breaking taboos. Bottoms like to explore feelings of being scared, overwhelmed, and out of control.

In my work as a sex educator, I've talked to thousands of people over the years, and some are big fans of playing rough but don't associate it with kink at all. It doesn't really matter what you call it. Rough sex is another kind of dominant/submissive role play where you can explore power, control, and surrender, and use intense physicality to push limits and break taboos. Rough sex can include BDSM activities like spanking, blindfolds, or bondage as well as smacking, pushing, grabbing, hair pulling, spitting, scratching, being held down, and face slapping. If these things sound fun to you, read on.

> *Rough sex tops get turned on by taking control of a partner's body, using physical force, and breaking taboos.*

Although some folks distinguish between rough sex and BDSM and others don't, what's most important is that the basic principles of kink should always be in play: consent, communication, negotiation, education, safety and risk reduction, and aftercare. Telling your partner, "I want it rough," just isn't specific enough. You need to negotiate, talk about what activities are off limits, and constantly check in about the degree of roughness that works for you. For example, some people love to be slapped in various places on their body, but being slapped in the face is too much for them. But if you are interested in being slapped in the face, think about what will make it sexy for you. Some love being spit on, but others find it degrading; where does it fall on your "Yes–No–Maybe" list? What about having your hair pulled? If you want your partner to grab you, push you, and generally "manhandle" you, talk about how you want that to feel.

> *You need to negotiate, talk about what activities are off limits, and constantly check in about the degree of roughness that works for you.*

You can learn rough sex skills, including proper techniques, parts of the body to avoid, as well as ways to reduce risk and avoid serious injury. (Yes, there are even classes on rough sex, as well as a fantastic chapter about it by Felice Shays in *The Ultimate Guide to Kink*.) If you're into hair pulling, you should get a good grip of the hair at the base of the scalp; you shouldn't ever pull the ends of the hair or yank someone's head by the hair. Slapping follows the rules of spanking and flogging: only smack fleshy parts like the butt, thighs, and upper back; avoid joints, bones, and internal organs. For the face, always hold someone's face with one hand and slap with the other, so they don't get whiplash. Some people like to be scratched, but make sure you communicate your boundaries: how do you feel about your skin being marked up or even bleeding? If you and your partner are interested in heavier kinds of impact play, like hitting, punching, or kicking, even if you're not a part of the local kink scene, investigate if there is a class or event that teaches you how to do them properly.

FIFTY ITEMS FOR YOUR TOY BAG

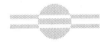

I've composed a list of fifty items for your toy bag—
some are for your actual stash of goodies, others are
for your metaphorical toy bag. Although there is a
lot of wonderful kinky gear available, know that a
sharp, creative mind is all you really need to have a
good time. So go forth and have one!

1. Consent
2. Communication
3. Honesty
4. "Yes–No–Maybe" list
5. A sense of humor

6. Compassion

7. Trust

8. Enthusiasm

9. An open mind

10. A commitment to adventure

11. Knowledge

12. Safewords

13. Condoms

14. Safer-sex supplies

15. Tissues

16. Hand sanitizer

17. Baby wipes

18. Lube

19. Nail clippers and a nail file

20. Notepad and pen

21. Bandanna

22. Silk scarf

23. Blindfold

24. Massage oil candle

25. Feather

26. Necktie

27. Gag

28. Collar

29. Leash
30. Bondage tape
31. Wrist and ankle cuffs
32. Carabiner clips
33. Rope
34. Safety scissors
35. Faux-fur covered paddle
36. Riding crop
37. Nipple clamps
38. Vibrator
39. Batteries or charger
40. Ben Wa balls
41. Dildo
42. Butt plug
43. Cock ring
44. Cane
45. Leather slapper
46. Clothespins
47. Athletic wrap and/or plastic wrap
48. Hood
49. Earplugs
50. Flogger

READING LIST

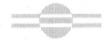

Nonfiction

Becoming a Slave, by Jack Rinella (Chicago: Rinella Editorial Services, 2005).

Different Loving: The World of Sexual Dominance and Submission, by Gloria Brame and William Brame (New York: Villard, 1996).

Leatherfolk: Radical Sex, People, Politics, and Practice, edited by Mark Thompson (Los Angeles: Daedalus Publishing, 2004).

Leathersex: A Guide for the Curious Outsider and the Serious Player, by Joseph W. Bean (Los

Angeles: Daedalus Publishing, 1994).

The Master's Manual: A Handbook of Erotic Dominance, by Jack Rinella (Los Angeles: Daedalus Publishing, 1994).

Miss Abernathy's Concise Slave Training Manual, by Christina Abernathy (Eugene, OR: Greenery Press, 1996).

The Mistress Manual: The Good Girl's Guide to Female Dominance, by Mistress Lorelei (Eugene, OR: Greenery Press, 2000).

The New Bottoming Book, by Dossie Easton and Janet Hardy (Eugene, OR: Greenery Press, 2001).

The New Topping Book, by Dossie Easton and Janet Hardy (Eugene, OR: Greenery Press, 2003).

Partners in Power: Living in Kinky Relationships, by Jack Rinella (Eugene, OR: Greenery Press, 2003).

Playing Well With Others: Your Field Guide to Discovering, Exploring, and Navigating the Kink, Leather and BDSM Communities, by Lee Harrington and Mollena Williams (Eugene, OR: Greenery Press, 2012).

Screw the Roses, Send Me the Thorns: The Romance and Sexual Sorcery of Sadomasochism, by Philip Miller and Molly Devon (Fairfield, CT: Mystic Rose Books, 1995).

The Seductive Art of Japanese Bondage, by Midori (Eugene, OR: Greenery Press, 2002).

Sensuous Magic: A Guide for Adventurous Couples, by Patrick Califia (Berkeley: Cleis Press, 2002).

Shibari You Can Use: Japanese Rope Bondage and Erotic Macramé, by Lee Harrington (New York: Mystic Productions Press, 2007).

SM 101: A Realistic Introduction, by Jay Wiseman (Eugene, OR: Greenery Press, 1998).

Two Knotty Boys Showing You the Ropes: A Step-by-Step, Illustrated Guide for Tying Sensual and Decorative Rope Bondage, by Two Knotty Boys (San Francisco: Green Candy Press, 2006).

The Ultimate Guide to Kink: BDSM, Role Play and the Erotic Edge, edited by Tristan Taormino (Berkeley: Cleis Press, 2012).

When Someone You Love Is Kinky, by Dossie Easton (Eugene, OR: Greenery Press, 2000).

Kinky Novels and Fiction Anthologies

◇◇◇◇◇◇◇

The Academy: Tales of the Marketplace, edited by Laura Antoniou (Cambridge, MA: Luster Editions, 2012).

Best Bondage Erotica, edited by Alison Tyler (Berkeley: Cleis Press, 2003).

Best Bondage Erotica 2013, edited by Rachel Kramer Bussel (Berkeley: Cleis Press, 2012).

Best Lesbian Bondage Erotica, edited by Tristan Taormino (Berkeley: Cleis Press, 2007).

Bound by Lust: Romantic Stories of Submission and Sensuality, edited by Shanna Germain (Berkeley: Cleis Press, 2012).

Carrie's Story: An Erotic S/M Novel, by Molly Weatherfield (Berkeley: Cleis Press, 2012).

Cheeky Spanking Stories, edited by Rachel Kramer Bussel (Berkeley: Cleis Press, 2012).

Hurts So Good: Unrestrained Erotica, edited by Alison Tyler (Berkeley: Cleis Press, 2011).

Macho Sluts, by Patrick Califia (Vancouver: Arsenal Pulp Press, 2009).

Making the Hook-Up: Edgy Sex with Soul, edited by Cole Riley (Berkeley: Cleis Press, 2010).

Mr. Benson, by John Preston (Berkeley: Cleis Press, 2004).

The Marketplace, by Laura Antoniou (Cambridge, MA: Circlet Press, 2010).

My Girlfriend Comes to the City and Beats Me Up, by Stephen Elliott (Berkeley: Cleis Press, 2006).

Please, Ma'am: Erotic Stories of Male Submission, edited by Rachel Kramer Bussel (Berkeley: Cleis Press, 2010).

Please, Sir: Erotic Stories of Female Submission, edited by Rachel Kramer Bussel (Berkeley: Cleis Press, 2010).

The Reunion, by Laura Antoniou (Fairfield, CT: Mystic Rose Books, 2003).

The Slave, by Laura Antoniou (Cambridge, MA: Circlet Press, 2011).

The Trainer, by Laura Antoniou (Cambridge, MA: Circlet Press, 2011).

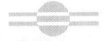

TRISTAN TAORMINO is an award-winning author, sex educator, speaker, filmmaker, and radio host. She is the author of seven books, including *The Secrets of Great G-Spot Orgasms and Female Ejaculation*, *The Ultimate Guide to Anal Sex for Women*, and *Opening Up: A Guide to Creating and Sustaining Open Relationships*. She is the editor of more than twenty-five anthologies including *The Ultimate Guide to Kink: BDSM, Role Play and the Erotic Edge*, and she is coeditor of *The Feminist Porn Book: The Politics of Producing Pleasure*. She was creator and series editor of the *Best Lesbian*

Erotica anthology series. Her books have sold over 500,000 copies and been translated into many languages. She's written for a multitude of publications from *Yale Journal of Law and Feminism* to *Penthouse*, and she served as editor of the magazine *On Our Backs*. She was a syndicated columnist for *The Village Voice* for nine and a half years and writes an advice column for *Taboo Magazine*.

Tristan is also the producer and host of Sex Out Loud, a weekly radio show on the VoiceAmerica Network. As the head of Smart Ass Productions, she has directed and produced twenty-four sex education and erotic films; she is currently an exclusive director for Vivid Entertainment. Her films have won more than a dozen awards, and she was the first female director to win the AVN Award for Best Gonzo Movie. Tristan and her work have been featured in over four hundred publications including *O: The Oprah Magazine*, *The New York Times*, *Redbook*, *Cosmopolitan*, *Glamour*, *Entertainment Weekly*, *Details*, *New York Magazine*, *Men's Health*, and *Playboy*. She has appeared on HBO's *Real Sex*, *The Howard Stern Show*, *Love-*

line, *Ricki Lake*, *Melissa Harris-Perry*, MTV, CNN, NBC, Oxygen, Fox News, the Discovery Channel, and on over a hundred radio shows.

Tristan lectures at top colleges and universities including Yale, Cornell, Princeton, Brown, Harvard, Columbia, Smith, Johns Hopkins, and UCLA, where she speaks on gay and lesbian issues, sexuality and gender, and feminism. She teaches sex and relationship workshops around the world. You can find her online at puckerup.com.

RACHEL KRAMER BUSSEL (rachelkramerbussel. com) is the editor of over fifty anthologies, including *Cheeky Spanking Stories; Serving Him: Sexy Stories of Submission; Please, Sir; Please, Ma'am; The Big Book of Orgasms; Baby Got Back: Anal Erotica; Flying High; Suite Encounters;* and the *Best Bondage Erotica* series. Follow her @raquelita on Twitter.

Many More Than Fifty Shades of Erotica

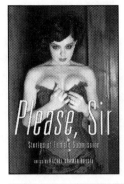

THE ULTIMATE GUIDES

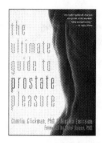

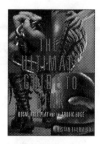

The Ultimate Guide to Prostate Pleasure Erotic Exploration for Men and Their Partners

Charlie Glickman, PhD and Aislinn Emirzian

$17.95, 6" x 9", 368 Pages,
Health/Sexuality,
ISBN: 978-1-57344-904-5,
Trade Paper, 32/case,
Rights: World

The Ultimate Guide to Kink BDSM, Role Play and the Erotic Edge

Tristan Taormino

$19.95, 6" x 9", 464 Pages,
Sexuality,
ISBN: 978-1-57344-779-9,
Trade Paper, 28/case,
Rights: World

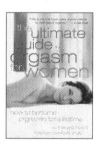

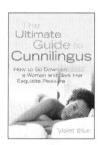

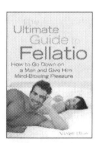

The Ultimate Guide to Orgasm for Women How to Become Orgasmic for a Lifetime

Mikaya Heart

$17.95, 6" x 9", 272 Pages,
Health/Sexuality,
ISBN: 978-1-57344-711-9,
Trade Paper, 40/case,
Rights: World

The Ultimate Guide to Cunnilingus How to Go Down on a Woman and Give Her Exquisite Pleasure

Violet Blue

$16.95, 6" x 9", 200 Pages,
Sexuality,
ISBN: 978-1-57344-387-6,
Trade Paper, 52/case,
Rights: World

The Ultimate Guide to Fellatio How to Go Down on a Man and Give Him Mind-Blowing Pleasure

Violet Blue

$16.95, 6" x 9", 272 Pages,
Sexuality,
ISBN: 978-1-57344-398-2,
Trade Paper, 36/case,
Rights: World

THE ULTIMATE GUIDES

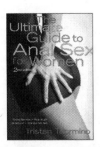

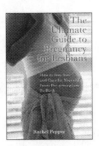

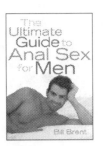

The Ultimate Guide to Anal Sex for Women
Tristan Taormino

$16.95, 6" x 9", 240 Pages,
Sexuality,
ISBN: 978-1-57344-221-3,
Trade Paper, 40/case,
Rights: World

The Ultimate Guide to Pregnancy for Lesbians
How to Stay Sane and Care for Yourself from Pre-conception Through Birth
Rachel Pepper

$17.95, 6" x 9", 288 Pages,
Health/Pregnancy & Childbirth,
ISBN: 978-1-57344-216-9,
Trade Paper, 36/case,
Rights: World

The Ultimate Guide to Anal Sex for Men
Bill Brent

$16.95, 6" x 9", 272 Pages,
Sexuality,
ISBN: 978-1-57344-121-6,
Trade Paper, 36/case,
Rights: World

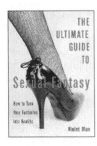

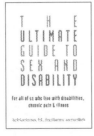

The Ultimate Guide to Sexual Fantasy
How to Turn Your Fantasies into Reality
Violet Blue

$15.95, 6" x 9", 272 Pages,
Sexuality,
ISBN: 978-1-57344-190-2,
Trade Paper, 32/case,
Rights: World

The Ultimate Guide to Sex and Disability
For All of Us Who Live with Disabilities, Chronic Pain and Illness
Miriam Kaufman, M.D., Cory Silverberg and Fran Odette

$18.95, 6" x 9", 360 Pages,
Health/Sexuality,
ISBN: 978-1-57344-304-3,
Trade Paper, 24/case,
Rights: World

"A welcome resource.... This book will be a worthwhile read for anyone who lives with a disability, loves someone with a disability, or simply wants to be better informed sexually."
—**Curve**

Classic Sex Guides

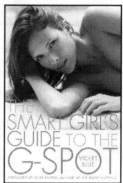

The Smart Girl's Guide to the G-Spot
Violet Blue

It's not a myth, it's a miracle, the G-spot, that powerhouse of female orgasm. With wit and panache, sex educator and bestselling writer Violet Blue helps readers master the sexual alphabet through G.
ISBN 978-1-57344-780-5 $14.95

The Smart Girl's Guide to Porn
Violet Blue

As seen on the Oprah Winfrey show!

Looking for authentic sex scenes? Thinking of sharing porn with a lover? Wonder which browser is safest for Internet porn surfing? *The Smart Girl's Guide to Porn* has the answers.
ISBN 978-1-57344-247-3 $14.95

The Adventurous Couple's Guide to Sex Toys
Violet Blue

Feeling adventurous? In this witty and well-informed consumer guide, bestselling author and sex educator Violet Blue shows couples how to choose and use sex toys to play and explore together—and have mind-blowing sex.
ISBN 978-1-57344-972-4 $14.95

The Adventurous Couple's Guide to Strap-On Sex
Violet Blue

"If you're seriously considering making it a part of your sexual repertoire, *The Adventurous Couple's Guide to Strap-On Sex* will give you all the advice you need to enjoy it in a safe and satisfying fashion." —*Forum UK*
ISBN 978-1-57344-278-7 $14.95

Seal It With a Kiss
Violet Blue

A great kiss can stop traffic, start a five-alarm fire, and feel like Times Square on New Year's Eve. Get your smooch on with all the different tricks and tips found in *Seal It with a Kiss*.
ISBN 978-1-57344-385-2 $12.95

Best Erotica Series

"Gets racier every year."—*San Francisco Bay Guardian*

Buy 4 books,
Get 1 FREE*

Best Women's Erotica 2013
Edited by Violet Blue
ISBN 978-1-57344-898-7 $15.95

Best Women's Erotica 2012
Edited by Violet Blue
ISBN 978-1-57344-755-3 $15.95

Best Women's Erotica 2011
Edited by Violet Blue
ISBN 978-1-57344-423-1 $15.95

Best Bondage Erotica 2013
Edited by Rachel Kramer Bussel
ISBN 978-1-57344-897-0 $15.95

Best Bondage Erotica 2012
Edited by Rachel Kramer Bussel
ISBN 978-1-57344-754-6 $15.95

Best Bondage Erotica 2011
Edited by Rachel Kramer Bussel
ISBN 978-1-57344-426-2 $15.95

Best Lesbian Erotica 2013
Edited by Kathleen Warnock.
Selected and introduced by
Jewelle Gomez.
ISBN 978-1-57344-896-3 $15.95

Best Lesbian Erotica 2012
Edited by Kathleen Warnock.
Selected and introduced by
Sinclair Sexsmith.
ISBN 978-1-57344-752-2 $15.95

Best Lesbian Erotica 2011
Edited by Kathleen Warnock.
Selected and introduced by Lea DeLaria.
ISBN 978-1-57344-425-5 $15.95

Best Gay Erotica 2013
Edited by Richard Labonté.
Selected and introduced by Paul Russell.
ISBN 978-1-57344-895-6 $15.95

Best Gay Erotica 2012
Edited by Richard Labonté.
Selected and introduced by
Larry Duplechan.
ISBN 978-1-57344-753-9 $15.95

Best Gay Erotica 2011
Edited by Richard Labonté.
Selected and introduced by
Kevin Killian.
ISBN 978-1-57344-424-8 $15.95

Best Fetish Erotica
Edited by Cara Bruce
ISBN 978-1-57344-355-5 $15.95

Best Bisexual Women's Erotica
Edited by Cara Bruce
ISBN 978-1-57344-320-3 $15.95

Best Lesbian Bondage Erotica
Edited by Tristan Taormino
ISBN 978-1-57344-287-9 $16.95

* Free book of equal or lesser value. Shipping and applicable sales tax extra.
Cleis Press • (800) 780-2279 • orders@cleispress.com
www.cleispress.com

Ordering is easy! Call us toll free or fax us to place your MC/VISA order.
You can also mail the order form below with payment to:
Cleis Press, 2246 Sixth St., Berkeley, CA 94710.

**Buy 4 books,
Get 1 FREE***

ORDER FORM

QTY	TITLE	PRICE
___	_____	_____
___	_____	_____
___	_____	_____
___	_____	_____
___	_____	_____
___	_____	_____
___	_____	_____
___	_____	_____

SUBTOTAL _____

SHIPPING _____

SALES TAX _____

TOTAL _____

Add $3.95 postage/handling for the first book ordered and $1.00 for each additional
book. Outside North America, please contact us for shipping rates. California resi-
dents add 9% sales tax. Payment in U.S. dollars only.

* Free book of equal or lesser value. Shipping and applicable sales tax extra.

**Cleis Press • Phone: (800) 780-2279 • Fax: (510) 845-8001
orders@cleispress.com • www.cleispress.com
You'll find more great books on our website**

Follow us on Twitter @cleispress • Friend/fan us on Facebook

Printed in the United States
By Bookmasters